DATE DUE

6/93/38	SEP 1 2 1997

GAYLORD

PRINTED IN U.S.A.

HOME CARE CONTROVERSY

Too Little, Too Late, Too Costly

Mary O'Neil Mundinger, R.N., Dr. P.H.

Columbia University School of Nursing
New York, New York

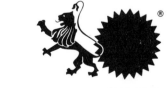

AN ASPEN PUBLICATION®

Aspen Systems Corporation
Rockville, Maryland
London
1983

Library of Congress Cataloging in Publication Data

Mundinger, Mary O'Neil
Home care controversy.

Includes bibliographies and index.
1. Aged—Home care—Government policy—United States.
2. Medicare. 3. Home care services—Government
policy—United States. 4. Aged—Home care—United
States. 5. Home care services—United States. I. Title.
[DNLM: 1. Delivery of health care—Economics.
2. Health insurance for aged and disabled, Title 18.
3. Home care services—Organization and administration.
4. Public health nursing. 5. Public
policy. WY115 M965h]
RA564.8.M86   1983   362.1'4'0973   83-11848
ISBN: 0-89443-883-2

Publisher: John Marozsan
Editorial Director: Darlene Como
Executive Managing Editor: Margot Raphael
Editorial Services: Jane Coyle
Printing and Manufacturing: Debbie Collins

Copyright © 1983 by Aspen Systems Corporation

Library of Congress Catalog Card Number 83-11848
ISBN: 0-89443-883-2

Printed in the United States of America

1 2 3 4 5

For Paul, Ann, Thomas, and Elizabeth

Table of Contents

Foreword

When President Johnson signed the amendments to the Social Security Act establishing Medicare and Medicaid in 1965, almost everyone believed that a great step had been taken toward providing adequate health care for the elderly of America. Despite initial reluctance, even the American Medical Association expected a positive outcome. And the care of the elderly has indeed been improved. Few foresaw, however, the pressure that increasing costs in hospitals and nursing homes would place on the whole structure of health care delivery, compounded as it has been by the amazing technological advances of the last eighteen years. In this volume, Dr. Mundinger traces the history of that legislation and its effects, particularly as they relate to home health services. The latter have now captured major attention because of the realization of the importance of keeping elderly patients out of high-cost facilities and at home for as long as possible.

As a result of her study of a home health agency in a suburban area of a northeastern state, Dr. Mundinger has been able to focus attention on the present failures of policy, shortcomings in the legislation itself, and on the serious problems posed by local application of the Medicare system of reimbursement. She addresses this by demonstrating the efforts health personnel—particularly public health nurses—make in attempting to bend regulations to meet the needs of patients and points out some solutions that modification of the law would allow.

It is clear from her findings that a new type of support system for the frail is needed in our society. Dr. Mundinger correctly concludes that a primary mistake is in trying to adapt the medical model of care to the needs of frail or disabled people when the real deficiency is in the areas of health education, social and psychological support, and prevention or reduction of disability. Physicians are rarely attuned to these community needs, whereas nurse practitioners and social workers are. Medicare designates physicians as leaders of the health delivery team although they are often remote from the point of delivery and not well schooled in dealing with problems encountered outside the hospitals and examining rooms.

The author has no intention of leaving physicians out of the picture, but recommends that nurses be responsible for nursing diagnosis and plan of management in the home. Physicians would continue to monitor the medical conditions that require treatment. This division of labor would be far more rational than the present arrangement and would foster better communication between physicians, nurses, and patients.

The primary aim of care in the home, as Dr. Mundinger points out, should be the prevention of institutionalization. Patients in danger of requiring hospitalization should be eligible for care in the home if that care can delay or prevent admission to high-cost facilities. Quite realistically, however, Dr. Mundinger emphasizes the fact that the requirements of some patients at home may be as expensive to meet as the costs of nursing home care or hospitalization. Expert judgment is required to determine the best setting for care and the dimensions of that care. She quite properly proposes congregate housing as a solution for many patients, especially those living alone.

The author's other recommendations are thoughtful and reflect her considerable experience as a professional nurse, teacher, and researcher. She makes a nice distinction between community-based and hospital-based home care services. She sees the latter as an extension of hospital services to patients discharged to recover from some medical condition. She feels that community-based services in the future might best be employed for the prevention of greater disability in those frail members of society who could benefit from support and protection.

Dr. Mundinger believes funding for home services, as presently organized, is quite unsatisfactory. She explores ways in which it could be made more effective and equitable without increasing the costs to unreasonable levels. Legislators and other policy-makers would do well to examine carefully her cogent suggestions, since the problems of the elderly and the number of frail and disabled in our population can only be expected to increase in the years ahead.

This book is a remarkably fine addition to the literature on health care delivery. It traces the history of efforts over the last few decades to meet the needs of people requiring community support; it reports the observations of a specific study of how home care is actually carried out and how it often fails to work in one section of the country; it concludes with an analysis of the problems still confronting us and recommended solutions for each. Everyone should benefit from reading this work—physicians, nurses, other health workers, and patients and potential patients as well.

George G. Reader, M.D.
Livingston Farrand Professor and
Chairman, Department of Public Health
Cornell University Medical College
August, 1983

Acknowledgments

Webster's Third New International dictionary makes the word *acknowledge* sound almost grudging—the first synonym is "admit" and the first meaning is given as: "to show by word or act that one has knowledge of and agrees to: concede to be right or true."

The acknowledgments for this book are hardly a grudging concession. They are a genuine "thank you," for in a very real sense this would not have been written without the guidance and assistance of many people.

The manuscript grew from the research for my doctoral dissertation, and if that had not been guided properly there would have been no book. The historical evolution of Medicare was written with the benefit of Dr. George Reader's incisive perspective of the American Medical Association's role in the development of the statute. Dr. Reader, one of the witnesses in the Congressional hearings on Medicare in the 1960s, even then was an articulate spokesman for the very issues only now being widely recognized by health policy analysts: that home care needs of the elderly are for health maintenance and disability prevention and that a medical framework is unnecessarily costly.

Analysis of Medicare policy was greatly enhanced with the generous assistance and advice of Prof. Frank Grad of the Columbia University School of Law. His genuine hospitality was complemented by his quick mind at work. Dr. Lowell Bellin, Professor of Public Health in the School of Public Health at Columbia and a member of my doctoral committee, has enriched my professional education for years, always asking the questions most likely to poke holes in a theory, pique my interest, or open new doors of inquiry. Dr. Lois Grau, also a committee member, added immeasurably to this project. Her own work on nursing home regulatory policy and her knowledgeable review were valuable throughout the research and the writing of the dissertation.

Most importantly, thanks to Dr. Melanie Dreher, who chaired my committee and was the major force and shaper of this study. She not only introduced me to qualitative research, she helped me develop it substantively as it related to home care issues. Her assistance was inspirational yet practical, and political as well as objective. Because of her intellectual and personal assistance, the study not only was fun, and productive, it also helped me develop skills for future projects.

Any family that puts up with a member doing doctoral research deserves praise and thanks; one that then allows the whole process to continue as the dissertation becomes a book earns far more. My husband, Paul, not only said it was a wonderful idea but supported it by asking questions that helped to develop the ideas more fully from the research. Our children, now young adults beginning to manage their own lives, honor my writing efforts by propping up my first book— *Autonomy in Nursing*—on their own college study desks—no small tribute. I hope this one goes there, too.

Two technical notes. First, in Chapters 5 and 6, all references to patients and their families are true and complete. Their names have been changed but their ethnicity has been preserved. Second, all demographic, economic, health status, and Medicare statistics used throughout the book, unless credited otherwise, are from projections for FY 1982, supplied by HCFA Office of Financial and Actuarial Analysis and from the *Health Care Financing Review* (Winter, 1981), published by the Health Care Financing Administration of the U.S. Department of Health and Human Services.

Mary O'Neil Mundinger, R.N., Dr. P.H.
August, 1983

Introduction

This book analyzes the structure and organization of home health services for the elderly and the failure of public policy in the delivery of that care.

Most home health services for the elderly are paid for by Medicare; if an individual also is indigent and lives in a state where home care is covered by Medicaid, that program may pick up some of the bill once the patient reaches the Medicare benefit limits. Medicare is just what it sounds like: medical care—or at least that is what federal policy meant it to be.

Where physicians are in charge, the care will be primarily medical in nature. Medicare was developed to maintain this direction. Health maintenance organizations (HMOs) are another example of the medical perspective. They are not really aimed at health maintenance so much as at achieving a more cost-effective method of treating episodic illnesses, particularly in substituting outpatient care for more expensive inpatient treatment.

Similarly, where high-technology care is available (e.g., in hospitals), it will be used more in relation to availability of the service than to patient needs. In nearly all health care settings, it is physicians who order the care, and they generally prescribe and provide the services they are most familiar with and perform the best. However, those may not necessarily be the services that patients need the most.

Since the mid-1970s, a better informed and more assertive patient population has made physician-directed care more subject to question. At the same time, the rise of professional awareness in the nursing profession has added the issue of its authority, which overlaps and sometimes conflicts with that of physicians, in the delivery of health care. These two factors have made it less likely that physician dominance in all health care desision making will continue to be as strong. Availability of services, source of payment, and perceived need by patients also have become influential in the determination of the health care they receive.

The Reagan administration pushed federal deregulation as its general overall policy but there are a number of reasons to expect and to advocate continued strong regulation in health care:

- The marketplace does not work well for health care. Consumers are not adequately informed as to how to choose the most effective or appropriate services.
- Consumers not only are inadequately prepared for those choices—they do not have the power to make them. It is the physician who orders drugs, determines admissions to hospitals, makes referrals, and who also can deny services deemed unnecessary. Therefore, the decision for utilization of specific health services remains primarily with the provider, not the consumer.
- Those with the most need for health services generally have the fewest dollars with which to purchase them. Scarce, expensive commodities, especially when highly subsidized with public funds, require a distribution and access system that assures equity. Without such regulation, services would be further restricted to the wealthy and to those who lived in areas where the providers chose to reside—hardly a system under which availability matches needs. Health service is publicly subsidized, expensive, and limited so it requires regulation.
- Regulation will continue to be necessary because of the increasingly restrictive nature of public financing for health care. Federal deregulation has forced the states to assume the responsibility for funding and rationing care, which requires them to develop regulations of their own to assure proper use of those public monies.

Because of the factors of absence of a true marketplace, the need to assure equity, and the need for accountability for decreasing resources, health care regulation will continue to be needed and strengthened.

The first broad federal health care legislation was Medicare and Medicaid in 1965 (Public Law 89-97). This was the product of a national concern about access, availability, and payment for health care for the elderly and the poor. By the late 1970s, because of success in increasing access and equity and because of a shrinking federal budget for health care, the focus of regulation switched to cost containment (Brook & Lohr, 1981).

The nation thus moved from a period of limited growth in health service availability to an era of cutbacks and trade-offs. In a time of retrenchment, protection of priority services became critically important. Priority services were those represented by the strongest power brokers—physicians and hospitals. A nationwide increase in interest in illness prevention, health maintenance, and active assumption of self-care health practices has emerged already.

Lack of resources to develop those areas, however, makes it less likely they will continue to grow. Even with evidence that preventive care can be cost effective and can raise the health status of populations served, those services are the first to go during cutbacks if the choice is between preventive services and acute medical care. The most powerful providers in health care delivery traditionally protect their status quo. Increased regulation, with its focus on cost containment, makes it difficult for innovative changes to occur unless they can be proved to be money savers.

The cost-containment regulatory structure and the highly medical nature of health services are factors that conflict in the delivery of home health services to the elderly. Such services usually are less costly than institutional care and are much more satisfying to the elderly as well (Somers & Bryant, 1975; U.S. Special Commission on Aging, 1974). Low cost and high satisfaction would seem to suggest these services should be developed fully.

In addition, the increased (and growing) number of elderly, and especially the very old (those over 80), makes home health services even more attractive in national planning. The decreasing availability of assistance by family members suggests that the public sector may well have to subsidize or substitute for home care that relatives traditionally used to supply. However, today's society regards health care primarily as medical care, so the medical framework has been superimposed on home health needs and services. Research shows that this medical structure and process of care is inappropriate (Trager, 1980; VanDyke & Brown, 1972; Vladeck, 1980). The home care needs of the elderly, even when they are convalescing from serious illness, are not medical in nature; rather, they call for nursing services and social assistance.

In a political atmosphere where cost containment is of prime importance and where the powerful faction composed of medical service providers insists on maintaining its primary share of resources, nursing does not have the strength or influence to fully meet its primary mission of providing illness prevention, health maintenance, and health promotion care.

Home care may be the most promising arena in which to demonstrate the value and cost effectiveness of nursing, particularly the health maintenance and disability prevention services. It is promising because it is a service destined to grow both because of need and because its costs are lower than institutional care. The true nature of those services, however, must be publicized widely if they are to be evaluated validly and used predictably. As it is, most professional preventive and maintenance services are being provided in home care under the guise of medical tasks.

Political necessity during the policy development phase has led to the development of home care as a medical service; however, professional nurses' subsequent implementation of that policy shows that different services are being delivered. The widespread manipulation of policy leads to health outcomes that never could have been obtained if the rules had been followed precisely. Yet because the true nature of the services is hidden, there is no way to measure outcomes of actual care accurately and no way to promote their value.

What is initially hidden becomes irretrievably lost: reimbursement policy cannot incorporate hidden services even when they may be responsible for advantageous outcomes. Manipulation of policy has only short-term rewards for patients or professionals, for ultimately policy will entrench only services that have been allowed, are documented, and therefore are supposed to be the causes of the actual outcomes. In times of cutbacks, those allowed services will be reduced further, making extra but hidden ones less possible.

If home health care policy is to be reformed, two kinds of data will be needed: (1) what services actually are delivered and for what purpose and (2) what the outcomes of those services are. Old ideas that health care is the same as medical care, and that outcomes must be measured in mortality or productivity, must be reexamined in terms of the population served. Home care is used mainly by the elderly. They are ill, yes, but generally their health problems cannot be cured, and their rehabilitation will not send them back to the work force. Instead, the value of home care must be seen as cost saving and life enriching for individuals whose health can be better maintained and preserved through professional and support services in the home.

The current role of physicians must change from overall direction of home care to direction of the medical aspects only, with a complementary role directing health-related nursing treatment. This is certainly not an antimedicine proposal, but a pronursing one that can focus accountability more appropriately where it belongs and can assure the elderly access to a full range of needed services.

This book begins by outlining the history and evolution of Medicare home health services. It addresses the defects and problems in this policy and links them to the political forces at work when the legislation was developed. This is followed by a discussion of a research study by the author that examines home care as actually given to 50 Medicare patients and analyzes the effectiveness of the policy and of professional decisions in the provision of home services. The final chapters look at current policy and make recommendations for the future.

REFERENCES

Brook, R., & Lohr, K. Quality of care assessment: Its role in the 80s. *American Journal of Public Health*, July 1981, *71*, 681-682.

P.L. 89-97, Social Security Amendments of 1965 (Medicare, Medicaid).

Somers, A., & Bryant, N. Home care: Much needed, much neglected. *Annals of Internal Medicine*, 1975, *82*(3).

Trager, B. *Home health care and national health policy*. New York: Hawthorne Press, 1980.

U.S. Special Commission on Aging. *Nursing home care in the U.S.: Failure in public policy.* Washington, D.C.: Author, 1974.

VanDyke, F., & Brown, V. Organized home care. *Inquiry*, June 1972, *9*, 3-16.

Vladeck, B. *Unloving care*. New York: Basic Books, Inc., 1980.

Chapter 1

Medicare: History and Intent

The passage of Medicare in 1965 had its beginnings in the English Poor Laws of more than 350 years ago. Those laws held communities responsible for the care of their needy citizens. They were extended to America during the 17th century. Publicly funded health care in this country therefore has existed since Colonial times.

Following the social and economic dislocations resulting from the Revolutionary War, communities found the needs of their citizens were greater than could be paid for by local resources so funding and direction of health services delivery became primarily a role of the state.

The federal government, being a government of limited powers, has primary authority for those areas listed in Section 8 of the Constitution. Article X of the Constitution makes it clear that the power over health matters is a prerogative of the states, not having been expressly designated a federal responsibility:

> The powers not delegated to the United States by the Consitution, nor prohibited by it to the States, are reserved to the States respectively, or to the people.

United States policy evolved to reflect the English Poor Laws after 1801, which directed local financial responsibility for only "indoor" relief, or institutionalization, as opposed to "outdoor" relief or subsidies that would enable individuals to remain independent (Rosenblum, 1979). During the 19th century the public health discipline grew rapidly. Local boards of health dated from Paul Revere's chairmanship in Massachusetts in 1799. By 1872 the American Public Health Association had been founded. That period was characterized by rapid growth of industry, railroads, and technology. There was more money and more leisure time; growth in urban populations rapidly outstripped the ability of cities to care for their inhabitants. It became clear that this population size and density created health needs that required the intervention of the state.

In the last half of the 19th century, public health agencies assumed the responsibility of protecting the public against disease, primarily through environmental tactics such as spraying for mosquitoes and establishing quarantines for communicable disease. By the 1900s the states had assumed care of the mentally ill and the blind while counties and cities had taken on the other "deserving poor" and the chronically ill, the feeble elderly, and the retarded.

EFFORTS IN THE 20TH CENTURY

The first effort for compulsory broad-based health insurance emerged as a national health insurance proposal in Theodore Roosevelt's Progressive Party platform in 1912. Similar proposals still were circulating in 1917, when the American Medical Association endorsed the idea for the first and only time, stating that to be against such a proposal "leaves the profession in a position of helplessness as the rising tide of social development sweeps over it" (Somers & Somers, 1967).

Publicly funded care continued to be mainly institutional, with poorhouses the feared and ultimate placement for many. In 1923 more than half the inhabitants of the poorhouses were over 65 and most were seriously disabled. The first half of the 20th century included both World Wars, with the Great Depression between them. Social welfare became an issue because of the poverty during the Depression and because prosperity from wartime employment gave impetus to social action programs. Government stepped in to provide the basic freedoms individuals could not provide for themselves. Differentiation of the "deserving" elderly from the (nondeserving) poor where they lived together in almshouses was one of the major factors that led to the establishment of Old Age Assistance, or cash subsidies to the elderly, under Title I of the Social Security Act of 1935 (P.L. 74-271) (Vladeck, 1980).

The Social Security Act of 1935 was proposed in the Senate by Senator Robert F. Wagner, Democrat of New York. His speech introducing the bill was passionate with the pain and pathos of the Great Depression from which the country was emerging (Senate, 1935). He declared the legislation was the natural consequence and the needed social action of that crisis. He added that the bill was a response to President Roosevelt's June 1934 speech calling for legislation to "cover the major social hazards of life."

In 1933 disabling sickness was 50 percent higher in families that had been affected most severely by the Depression, and in 1935, for the first time in decades, the death rate in large cities was higher than the previous year (Senate, 1935). Clearly the Depression had brought health care needs, as well as other economic problems, to the fore. The initial SSA bill proposed health insurance benefits for the elderly but that was withdrawn because of the strong opposition from the medical profession. The final bill added a small monthly increment ($30) to benefit checks if needed for health care but provided no restrictions as to how that money could be used. Many of the same legislators who agreed to that withdrawal of medical insurance coverage spent the next 30 years trying to put it back in. This was the nation's first instance of federally funded "outdoor" relief. It gave credence to the concept that poverty resulted from inadequate income and not from deficits in character or imprudent spending (Vladeck, 1980).

The cash subsidies were established as federal grants-in-aid to the states to be disbursed as means-tested (need-based) old age pensions. This program built on and strengthened pension programs in many of the states. The subsidies were forbidden to inmates of public institutions (almshouses) who already were being subsidized with public funds. However, the promise of pensions if they got out could do little to assist the elderly infirm in leaving the almshouses since money was only part of their need. They also required supportive health care—and it was unavailable to the noninstitutionalized. Therefore, only the able elderly could leave the almshouses, claim their pensions, and survive on their own.

Elderly persons who became frail and in need of assistance after the old age assistance checks became available, however, no longer were forced to enter almshouses but instead could choose nursing homes for which they could pay with their pensions. The system of providing only institutional care for disability remained; the Social Security Act simply changed the scene from almshouse to nursing home and the method from charity care to payment by check.

THE YEARS OF CHANGES

During the next 15 to 20 years legislation reflected the growing acceptance of nursing homes as medical facilities. The Social Security Act was amended in 1950 (P.L. 81-734) to allow cash subsidies to residents of public medical facilities and the 1946 Hill-Burton Act (P.L. 79-725), known mainly as a funding source for hospital construction, was amended to include nursing home construction "in conjunction with a hospital." These changes are important for two reasons: (1) welfare and health care were becoming interwoven although Congress always had intended to keep them separate and (2) national health policy continued to limit publicly funded treatment to institutions, not in-home care.

Two years after the passage of the Social Security Act a survey showed that 90 percent of the population had inadequate medical care. That same year in a proposal dubbed "professional birth control" the AMA led a successful campaign for medical schools to decrease the number of entering students, creating a physician shortage so that doctors' salaries would rise. The AMA also fought federal health insurance programs, contending that "any system of medicine that relieves the recipient of direct contribution for medical care will lower his responsibility for his own health" (Harris, 1966).

During World War II many young men were found to be medically unacceptable for military service, suffering from disabilities that could have been treated if care had been available. Those who did qualify for service found out what it was like to have adequate medical care available on demand when needed without cost. It was this generation that would support federally funded health insurance 20 years later.

During the 1940s and 1950s, numerous bills were submitted in Congress proposing various forms of comprehensive national health insurance. President Roosevelt's State of the Union message in 1944 included his commitment to the "right to adequate medical care and the opportunity to achieve and enjoy good health." A year later President Truman proposed comprehensive national prepaid health insurance through Social Security. Although Senator Robert A. Taft, Republican of Ohio, in 1946 proposed a health insurance plan limited to the poor, the mood of the country already was moving toward federal efforts to provide medical care as a universal "right" and not simply as a national responsibility toward the needy; almost all plans were to be financed through "earnings" in the Social Security program. In 1950 Congress amended the Social Security Act to give federal grants to the states for direct payment to health care providers for the treatment of welfare beneficiaries (P.L. 81-734). This created an administrative framework for welfare medical care that many wanted to use as a basis for developing a program of health care for all Social Security beneficiaries.

President Eisenhower, who received free, federally financed health care most of his life, and who therefore could have been a strong, knowledgeable advocate for national health insurance, favored instead a system of broader private coverage, with federal insurance against heavy losses. During 1956 alone, however, four bills were introduced in Congress for federally funded health insurance for Social Security beneficiaries. House Ways and Means Committee hearings on the bills, plus a report from the Senate Subcommittee on Aging, made it clear that the number one concern of the aged was the cost of health care. None of these bills passed, however.

There still were efforts to provide coverage only for the needy; these were described as reflecting the power of the AMA lobby and the public concern for the cost of a program that would provide universal coverage. The AMA's lower opposition to a need-only program was ascribed to the fact that it would not interfere with the status of physicians' direction in care given and fees charged and would insure them against loss of money from nonpayment by their poor patients. Universal coverage, however, was called socialized medicine and was seen by physicians as a threat to the very core of the medical practice system. The other reason that only the needy were considered in some proposals was the difference in cost between that reduced program and universal coverage.

THE FIRST MAJOR STEP: KERR-MILLS

During the 1960 presidential campaign Senator John F. Kennedy backed a proposal very much like the ultimate Medicare program: universal coverage for all elderly financed through Social Security. His opponent, Vice President Richard M. Nixon, backed a program of federal assistance to voluntary insurance programs. Both proposals lost and instead Medical Assistance to the Aged (MAA), the Kerr-Mills bill, was passed that year.

This provided federal grants-in-aid to the states, with the federal contribution based inversely on the per capita income of the state. These funds were used by the states to provide health care for the "medically indigent"—elderly persons who were not poor enough for welfare but, because of their medical bills, needed assistance. The program was voluntary, with no federal ceiling on contributions and with states determining eligibility. Even with these broad incentives for the states, only 14 chose to participate in the first year of the program. (Kerr-Mills lasted only through fiscal year 1966.) The means test was distasteful because it not only called upon the elderly to claim inability to pay their medical bills but also required their children to claim inability to pay for their parents' health care. The elderly would not apply with those double burdens on their pride.

The states that did take advantage of MAA funds were mainly those that already had well-developed medical services for the needy and that therefore were grateful to have federal assistance with those costs. MAA thus served to underwrite care in the least needy states. In states where needs were greater and resources less, even MAA assistance was not sufficient to implement such a program.

When Kennedy became president he continued his long-standing commitment to health care for the aged. Just ten days into his presidency he sent a special message to Congress outlining specific coverage in a health insurance program for the elderly. The bill failed mainly because of the organized efforts of the AMA, which was particularly concerned with the lack of "freedom of choice" for patients and with what it regarded as inadequate physician input in the proposed utilization review process.

That same year a survey showed that every country with a government-financed health care system was superior to the United States in longevity and infant mortality rates and that 60 percent of the doctors and 90 percent of the patients in those countries were satisfied with the system (Harris, 1966).

Voluntary health insurance and public funds each paid 20 percent of the costs of health care in the United States in the early 1960s. The care that was being paid for was expensive crisis illness treatment. People tended to try to meet their own expenses and applied for welfare help only when they became "very sick and very broke" (Piore, 1968). There was little preventive or maintenance care. The 1960s, a time of economic well-being, were similar to the awakening after the Depression; each served to develop a climate conducive to optimum social progress.

The same ideals that had spawned the Social Security Act served to engender Medicare and Medicaid three decades later. A health policy expert in 1965 wrote that the "good times in the sixties should give us the needed policies and programs for security of health services" and that the country had a "rising ability and readiness to pay for it" (Falk, 1965).

Medical care was becoming accepted as a necessity and a right, and rights belong to everyone. Increased income and an improved standard of living made the list of "necessities" broader. Since expensive commodities (e.g., medical care) are not distributed equally, they should be financed through public funds to assure equity. This is even more true for the aged, who not only have less income but also have greater need. This argument by a health economist (Scitovsky, 1964) was the basic reason for beginning first with the aged in a program of federally financed health care.

Most of the health policy literature in the early sixties agreed on the need for federal assistance in providing catastrophic coverage. The poor and the elderly were the two groups singled out as most in need of that help; often, they were the same group. By the mid-1960s, the annual incomes of two-thirds of those over 65 averaged $1,000 and the other third $3,000. While trying to subsist on these meager amounts, their medical bills were two and a half times those of the rest of the population (Harris, 1966). Health policy literature outlined the "future" need for a national health system but it was not a popular proposal for the sixties.

THE POWER OF THE PROVIDERS

The country was not in a completely altruistic mood, however; what was good for the elderly and poor also was good for the providers. The powerful physician and hospital groups were eager to be assured payment from those who were finding it increasingly difficult to meet their medical bills. A witness in the House Ways and Means Committee hearings on an early version of the Medicare bill stated in 1961 that "the aged can't pay their health care bills. They go on public welfare and accentuate the financial difficulties of hospitals" (House, 1961).

Not only were medical costs rising, the number of elderly also was increasing. They lived on fixed incomes and were beneficiaries of care that was increasing in complexity and in cost. Compounding the payment problem for providers was the finding in a 1965 survey that voluntary contributions for public health services were dropping, state expenditures were necessarily growing to meet the deficit, and the need for public sector financing of health care was becoming more of an issue (Freeman & Levenson, 1965).

THE LEGISLATION EVOLVES

A Gallup poll in the early 1960s showed that two-thirds of those responding were willing to increase their Social Security payments in order to fund federal health care for the elderly. A number of bills on the subject went to Congress early in Kennedy's presidency, although none was passed. In 1964, Senator Jacob Javits, Republican of New York, introduced legislation much like what became the final Medicare law, and although both the House and the Senate passed the bill in slightly different form, they could not agree on a final version.

Another grander and more liberal version was submitted by Representative John W. Byrnes, Republican of Wisconsin, and although it predictably failed, it served a political purpose for Representative Wilbur Mills, Democrat of Arkansas, chairman of the House Ways and Means Committee. Mills, coauthor of the Kerr-Mills MAA legislation of 1960, had seen the problems and deficits in that law's poor utilization and wanted coverage for the poor that would not include a means test for the relatives of the poor. The Byrnes bill made Mills' liberalized version of MAA less distasteful to the AMA. In addition, Mills had swung from being a major critic of federally funded health insurance to becoming its chief architect. As chairman, he was in a position to formulate the House version of health legislation. He envisioned a "layer cake" approach, with health care for the elderly in two layers—hospital care and physician care—with the third layer being care for the poor, a "repair" of Kerr-Mills.

While the AMA fought every effort to pass legislation for universal coverage of the elderly, it did agree to a system of payment that would require patients to submit to a means test. The AMA held that care that was subsidized as a "right" could only mean socialized medicine down the road, but government payment for previously endured charity care was acceptable.

The Byrnes bill, which would have provided far more benefits than others and under a government subsidy, brought a counterproposal from the AMA: Eldercare. Eldercare was a "liberalization" of Kerr-Mills in that it covered the indigent elderly, especially for payment of physicians' bills. One anti-AMA physician witness called Eldercare a "key to the U.S. Treasury" for physicians to assure payment for their services to the poor. Mills, instead of accepting Eldercare in lieu of coverage that did not involve a means test for the elderly, combined the two into what became Medicare and Medicaid.

The hearings on Medicare and Medicaid were held by the Congressional committees most involved in the economic, rather than health, aspects of the legislation: the Senate Finance Committee and the House Ways and Means Committee. Much of the testimony before each committee dwelt on two issues: (1) whether the health insurance was to cover only the needy and (2) where the revenues would come from. Congressional hearings, while providing a forum for generating ideas on proposed legislation, also are a vehicle for putting into the record the intent of the measure.

Clearly the overriding intent of this bill was to assist in paying medical bills of the elderly and the poor. However, it also impacted on the means test and the source of financing, and these intents are apparent in the hearing records. One was, in the 1960s era of racial progress, to abolish second-class segregated care; the second was to initiate a program that could be expanded into a national health insurance system. These goals were accomplished in Mills's compromise between the Byrnes and AMA versions that produced the final Medicare and Medicaid bills. Until that time, bills submitted had been for either means-tested coverage or universal coverage. Mills was able to negotiate a combination; means-tested coverage for those under age 65, and universal for those over 65.

Two concerns were apparent throughout the legislative process: (1) whether the AMA would defeat the proposals and (2) whether there might not be adequate service capacity for the large, newly enfranchised populace. These issues led to inclusion of liberal payments to providers and to the introductory clause that the government did not intend to interfere in the practice of medicine.

The aim of the legislation—federal health insurance coverage for the elderly and the poor—was politically favorable because the care providers, a powerful lobby, had much to benefit from such a law since it would assure them payment from the two groups that could not meet their bills. The main stumbling block, from the providers' standpoint, was the scope of coverage and financing base. If all of the elderly were covered (including those able to fund their own care) the providers would have had less to gain; universal coverage, to them, spelled socialized medicine.

The financing base for universal coverage already had a precedent: the Social Security system. Roosevelt had been adamant that the 1935 pension system be financed by deductions from both employers and employees, making the benefit an "earned right" and not charity. Proponents of universal health care coverage for the elderly in 1965 continued that belief: that funds for such a program also should come from those "earned" dollars of Social Security deductions from income. If a universal program were to be funded, instead, through general revenues, it would be seen as government subsidized care that quickly could become universal coverage for everyone.

THE THREE CORNERSTONES

The proposal before Congress in 1964 and 1965 (which eventually passed) provided three things:

1. universal coverage for hospital care for the elderly financed through payroll deductions under Social Security

2. optional supplementary insurance for physicians' services that would be financed by general revenues and a monthly individual premium
3. coverage for the poor funded by state and federal revenues, with state-determined eligibility and scope of services.

The AMA was particularly leery of the proposal that would allow supplementary coverage to be financed by individual premiums and general revenues. Mahlon Eubank, director of the Social Insurance Department of the New York State Commerce and Industry Association, testified on the medical and insurance industry concerns. He said voluntary premium-based insurance "puts the government in the insurance business. This would be merely a prelude to the government takeover of health insurance for people under 65. Within the near future individuals under 65 who will be subject to increased payroll and income taxes could demand the same right to buy their insurance on an optional basis and socialized medicine might well result" (House, 1964, p. 362).

Obviously such concerns could be resolved only by building in benefits for physicians and the insurance industry. This emerged in the provision that the only premium-based care was specifically for the coverage of physicians' bills, and already established private insurance companies were to be utilized as "intermediaries" and "carriers" (processors of claims) for the government program.

Framers of the legislation needed to assure not only that physicians and other providers would not block the legislation but equally important that they would participate in providing care to the newly entitled population. Therefore, statutory benefits for providers went further than statements of noninterference in the care process and in development of a funding base that was least likely to lead to socialized medicine. In addition, the statute provided for reimbursement methods that were uniquely advantageous to providers and to participating insurance companies.

These are described in detail in Chapter 3, on Medicare problems, but it is important to remember here that those decisions were seen as politically necessary in order to assure adequate access for Medicare beneficiaries. Other than reimbursement advantages and the clause that the bill included no intent for governmental intervention in the practice of medicine, there were additional concessions to physicians in order to gain their support:

1. Physician participation in Medicare would be voluntary.
2. Physicians would be in charge of utilization review activities, which were attempts to assure adequacy and appropriateness of care reimbursed under Medicare. Ironically, this placed physicians in the position of monitoring their own practice.
3. Physician certification would be required for all Medicare services, including nursing home and home health services as well as hospitalization.

The aim of abolishing second-class care also required concessions and benefits for providers. The elderly, the poor, and blacks often received care that was different from that provided to the higher income white population before 1965, particularly in the South (Feder, 1977). This resulted in part from the way institutions saw their responsibilities toward charity patients and in part from deeply rooted racial inequities. The Medicare legislation included two requirements that made this division of care less likely:

1. No hospital that segregated patients could participate in the Medicare program, meaning it could not receive reimbursement for the care of Medicare-eligible patients.
2. Only (and all) care delivered to Medicare beneficiaries could be reimbursed. This effectively removed the incentive to deliver substandard care because whatever was delivered was what would be reimbursed.

THE ROOTS OF COMPROMISE

The aim of providing a model for national health insurance in the future was accomplished through establishing a program of universal (nonmeans-tested) care and by protecting and promoting benefits for providers. Although the AMA was dead set against universal federal coverage for any group, it faced a society that generally was strongly interested in racial equality and social progress. To be against health care for the elderly was an unpopular stance in 1965. The AMA position that only the needy elderly should be covered also was unpopular because it was the antithesis of the liberal ideology then prevalent in the country. One witness in a Congressional hearing observed: "The use of a means test . . . automatically divides the citizens into two groups—the successful and the unsuccessful" (House, 1964, p. 289).

The AMA thus discerned that its stance in favor of means-tested coverage was unacceptable to Congress. That, along with the financial and professional incentives proposed, led to the AMA's eventual acceptance of Medicare. Its opposition had been costly: it had spent $23 million in 1965 alone and $50 million in all in its long campaign (Harris, 1966).

Another group was strongly in favor of the broad-based proposal and, though less visible than the medical community, had political strength in promoting the legislation: organized labor. The House hearings made it clear that Medicare was attractive to labor for two major reasons:

1. Funding medical insurance for retired workers meant that hospital care would become one of the pension benefits at least partially financed by employer deductions.

2. Guaranteed dependable health care for the elderly made it more likely that older workers would be able to retire, thereby opening employment opportunities for younger job aspirants.

Senator Albert Gore, Democrat of Tennessee, in the hearings on that chamber's bill, stated: "We want to encourage and promote retirement of people at age 65 in order to make way for employment possibilities for the teeming millions of youngsters coming out of our high schools and colleges" (Senate, 1964, p. 118).

The political maneuvering in Congress, particularly by Mills, the financial incentives for providers, and the broad-based nationwide support for social progress and equity made passage of Medicare possible in 1965. Although the achievement was an enormous one, hindsight indicates that Congress and the nation might have been ready to accept an even broader program.

President Kennedy, always a strong backer of health care for the aged, built it into his "New Frontier" programs. When he was assassinated in 1963, the nation rallied around President Johnson's commitment to passing what would be a legislative legacy to Kennedy's service. In 1964, while the Medicare bill was still in Congressional hearings, Johnson was elected president in a landslide. He not only saw this as a mandate to continue social legislation in his own framework, "The Great Society," he also was responding to an important increase in the number of elderly voters: in the 1964 election, 22 percent of the voters were over age 60. In addition to Johnson, 36 new liberal members of Congress were elected, further enhancing the possibility that Congress would approve social legislation such as medical care.

ACHIEVEMENT AND IMPLEMENTATION

Medicare was passed in the summer of 1965 and went into effect July 1, 1966. Continuing concerns were apparent about whether the nation's hospitals would be able to care for the newly insured elderly, who some expected to appear in droves at the doors of the institutions on that day. In fact, the first day of implementation was carefully chosen to be on a weekend and preceding the Fourth of July holiday, both of which would cause lower than normal hospital occupancy, thereby making available the additional beds that would be needed by the Medicare beneficiaries.

The front page of *The New York Times* on the first day of Medicare carried the headline shown in Exhibit 1-1.

The legislation was a predictable follower of the original Social Security Act of three decades earlier and was passed in the same economic upswing and period of social consciousness as its predecessor. It was the right idea at the right time.

Exhibit 1-1 A Memorable Headline

MEDICARE STARTS TODAY; 17 MILLION SIGNED

Smooth Beginning Expected;
Hospitals with 92% of
Beds Are Qualified

CHECK ON HOSPITAL OCCUPANCY

The social climate was right, with a liberal Democratic Congress and president, and a national interest in civil rights. The financial needs of both the elderly and the hospitals were apparent. Medicare therefore was passed as a reflection of this national mood.

REFERENCES

Falk, I.S. Medical care and social policy. *American Journal of Public Health,* April 1965, 522-527.

Feder, J. Medicare implementation and the policy process. *Journal of Health Policy, Politics & Law,* Summer 1977, *3*(3), 173-189.

Freeman, V., & Levenson, G. Income and expenditures in public health nursing agencies. *Nursing Outlook,* March 1965.

Harris, R. *A sacred trust.* New York: New American Library, 1966.

Piore, N. Rationalizing the mix of public and private expenditures in health. *Milbank Memorial Fund Quarterly,* January 1968, 161-170.

P.L. 79-725, Hill-Burton Act of 1946.

P.L. 74-271, Social Security Act of 1935.

P.L. 81-734, Social Security Act of 1950.

Medical Assistance to the Aged (1960).

Rosenblum, R. *The evolution of federal health care financing programs for the aged.* Unpublished doctoral dissertation, Columbia University, 1979.

Scitovsky, F. Medicare care—A necessity? in *Economics of Health and Medical Care*. Ann Arbor, Mich.: University of Michigan Press, 1964.

Somers, A., & Somers, H. *Medicare and the hospitals: Issues and prospects*. Washington, D.C.: The Brookings Institution, 1967.

U.S., Congress, House, Committee on Ways and Means, Hearings on H.R. 4222, 87th Cong., 1st sess., 1961.

U.S., Congress, Senate, Committee on Finance, Hearings on S.6675, 88th Cong., 2d sess., 1964.

U.S., Congress, Senate, Committee on Finance, Hearings on S.1130, 74th Cong., 1st sess., 1935.

Vladeck, B. *Unloving care*. New York: Basic Books, Inc., 1980.

Chapter 2

Medicare: The First 17 Years

There were more than 26 million people over the age of 65 in the United States as of the end of 1980. They accounted for 11 percent of the total population. Nearly all, plus another 3 million disabled, were covered by Medicare. In FY 1982 $321 billion was spent in the United States for health care, nearly 10.4 percent of the gross national product (GNP). Health care expenditures have been claiming an ever-increasing percentage of the GNP since Medicare began but the growth became alarmingly rapid in 1979, with the rise in such costs at a rate greater than that of the GNP.

The increase can be linked to Medicare in major ways. The advance in all health care expenditures in 1980 was more than 11.8 percent; the Medicare increases when measured alone were up more than 16 percent. Medicare costs were therefore rising 40 percent faster (HCFA Office of Financial and Actuarial Analysis, personal communication). From the operational start of Medicare in 1966 through 1980 the health care expenditure growth has been attributed to prices (up 58 percent), population (up 9 percent), and the number and intensity of services (up 34 percent) (HCFA, Spring 1981). The majority of the increases in price and intensity of services nationwide has been in hospital care, where Medicare spends the greatest amount of dollars on beneficiaries. In 1982 public funds paid for more than 42 percent of all health care expenditures; of that, more than a third went for personal care services to Medicare beneficiaries.

Table 2-1 shows the increased percentage of GNP spent for health care since 1929, and demonstrates the precipitous increases since Medicare.

The dollar amounts are equally staggering. In 1982 the entire nation (both private and government sectors) spent $321 billion on health care, more than seven times as much money as in 1965 ($41.5 billion). Even so, the private sector is still paying more than half the nation's health care bills. Home health services are a very minor part of Medicare expenditures, reaching a high in 1982 of 2.6 percent of all of its dollars spent, or $1.25 billion. Medicare dollars are accounted for in

Table 2-1 Spending on Health Care: Its Share of Gross National Product

Year	GNP in Billions of Dollars	Health Care Percent of GNP	Dollar Amount for Health Care in Billions
1929	$ 103	3.5	$ 3.6
1940	$ 100	4.0	$ 4
1950	$ 287	4.4	$ 12.6
1955	$ 400	4.4	$ 17.6
1960	$ 507	5.3	$ 26.8
1965	$ 691	6.0	$ 41.5
1970	$ 993	7.5	$ 74.4
1975	$1549	8.6	$133
1980	$2626	9.4	$247
1981	$2859	9.6	$274
1982	$3086	10.4	$321

Source: HCFA.

four major categories: hospital care, nursing home care, physicians' services, and "other personal health expenditures." Home health is included in the last category and in hospital care if the certified home health agency is hospital based.

The majority of home health care clients are over 65—in many states, nearly 75 percent of them. The most common medical diagnoses of home care patients are circulatory disease, diabetes, and cancer. Half of the severely disabled persons in this country are over 65 and 40 percent of all the elderly are disabled to some degree (DHEW, 1979). Disabilities also are present in the majority of home health clients. Activities of daily living, functional status, and mental condition are major problems for the aged receiving home care. For instance, in one study 20 percent of the patients were not alert sometimes, 9 percent were depressed, 60 percent needed help bathing or walking, and nearly 90 percent needed household assistance (HCA, 1979).

The kinds of home care the elderly need, and their illnesses, changed little during Medicare's first 17 years. Hospital care remains the most expensive component. What has changed is the growth, both actual and relative, of the size of the aged sector in the U.S. population. There are far more elderly (over 65) and very old elderly (over 75) than in 1965, and both groups continue to grow in size.

Between 1960-1970 Americans over age 65 increased by 21 percent, as compared with a 13 percent increase for the under age 65 group. Continuing increase in the elderly population is projected in Table 2-2. The potential need for comprehensive health services for a large elderly population, plus the enormous cost

Table 2-2 Projected Increase in the Elderly Population

Year	65+	75+
1900	4%	
1980	10.8%	4.2%
1990	11.5%	4.6%
2000	13.1%	4.9%

Source: Carl Pegels, *Health care and the elderly.* Rockville, Md.: Aspen Systems, 1981, pp. 1-2, 11-12.

increases in the program, both are responsible for the statutory and regulatory changes reflected in Medicare's history. That history is detailed next in terms of the original statute, the amendments, and the regulations.

THE STATUTE

Medicare is Title XVIII of the Social Security Act, P.L. 89-97, the Social Security Amendments of 1965. It creates a federally financed health insurance program for the over-65 population covered by Social Security or the Railroad Retirement program. It essentially is a bill-paying plan, financed by Social Security taxes for hospital coverage and general revenues and individual premiums for supplementary coverage. The funding sources have not changed but eligibility has been broadened to include nearly all over-65 persons, plus the disabled and ESRD (end stage renal disease) patients.

Medicare was administered initially by the Bureau of Insurance in the Department of Health, Education, and Welfare (HEW) and, since 1978, by the new Health Care Financing Administration, now in HEW's successor, the Department of Health and Human Services (HHS). The statute authorizes the secretary of HEW (now HHS) to establish and administer regulations to govern Medicare. The act has been amended every year or two to authorize either a higher wage base or an increase in individual premiums in order to fund the program adequately (1977 amendments in particular addressed the inadequate funding base).

Medicare has two distinct parts, A and B. Part A is for hospital or posthospital costs and is funded by Social Security taxes from employees, employers, and the self-employed. Part B is funded mainly through general revenues and by monthly individual premiums. It offers supplementary coverage to Part A such as payment for physician fees and added home health services. Participation in Part B is voluntary, although approximately 97 percent of those under Part A have both.

Home health services are not subject to copayment or deductibles by patients, and are reimbursed at 100 percent of reimbursable cost to providers. A number of "competitive" proposals for cost-sharing with patients have been proposed in Congress since 1982, and increasingly restrictive cost-caps limit agency cost reimbursement. Home care is available to patients posthospitalization or in lieu of hospitalization with no limit on the number of visits. Cost limitation is achieved in the following ways: (1) care is allowed only for an acute spell of illness, and (2) care is carefully audited after the first few weeks of service to assure continuing quality of care.

Home Services Defined

Home health services are defined in the act as skilled, intermittent, part-time services provided under a physician's written direction and plan of care, in the residence of the homebound client. The skilled services may be those of a registered nurse, physical therapist, or speech therapist and may include a home health aide, medical social worker, or occupational therapist. The services must be related to the medical diagnosis for which the initial care was instituted and must be provided under the auspices of a certified home health agency.

Home health services under both Medicare parts are subject to claims processing by intermediaries—private insurance companies approved by Medicare and bid for by the voluntary home health agencies and by hospitals and nursing homes as their claims processors. Other certified home health agencies must use the Division of Direct Reimbursement in the Medicare offices as their intermediary. The role of the intermediary is to assure proper disbursement of Medicare money and to assist agencies and institutions in efficient and appropriate delivery of services. Blue Cross is the major intermediary.

Carriers are the claims processors for other services, such as physicians; the major carrier is Blue Shield. Home health services are more like those of physicians than those of hospitals in that they consist of noninstitutional aid provided by single caregivers, but claims are under the institutional review of intermediaries, not carriers. Carriers have the same functions as intermediaries for Medicare except that the latter determine reimbursement on "reasonable cost" and carriers use "customary and prevailing charges." Both of these methodologies are spelled out in the regulations.

Home Health Agencies Defined

Home health agencies are defined as public or private entities primarily engaged in providing skilled nursing services as well as physical and speech therapy. The agencies, to be certified for participation in Medicare, also must have direct or contract arrangements for the provision of occupational therapy, medical social services, and home health aides. The agencies also must abide by Medicare eligibility regulations; adopt policies, claims procedures, and recordkeeping in accordance with regulations; and develop active committees, including professional advisory, physicians' advisory, utilization review, and quality assurance.

Section 1862 of the statute limits eligibility under both Parts A and B to "treatment of *illness* or *injury* or to *improve* the function of a malformed body member" (emphasis added). This focus on the medical curative process is evidence that Medicare home health services were not intended to be preventive or for health maintenance.

Under Part A, patients can receive home health services only for the condition for which they were hospitalized; under Part B, which has no prior hospitalization requirement, home health care is limited to only those services available in a hospital. In addition, the medical focus requires that home care beneficiaries be under the care of a physician and that the treatment they receive must be established, planned, and reviewed by the doctor.

Home health agencies, through their broad and sophisticated scope of services available, their complex recordkeeping and committee structure, and their change in service function to short-term, acute care convalescence, became a new entity on the home care scene. They differed significantly from their predecessors, which were small voluntary nursing agencies that provided home nursing care, some of the patients being convalescent but many permanently disabled or in need of long-term support.

Financial Incentives Omitted

Home health agencies came into being, on paper, in the Medicare act and Congress presumed that the small visiting nurse agencies would simply add on the services and develop the organizational systems in order to become home health agencies. It also was assumed that since no new buildings were needed (as there are with hospitals or nursing homes), development of the increased service delivery would not require any financial assistance.

Where hospitals and nursing homes were given preferential mortgage availability at federally subsidized interest rates, provided with cost-plus reimbursement, allowed to claim depreciation on capital equipment that had been totally federally financed, and in many other ways had financial incentives to develop service capability for Medicare beneficiaries, home health agencies received nothing. The majority of federal funding for home health services predated Medicare. From 1968 to 1975 the only federal grants were for paraprofessional training and for some additional service development funded under the Older Americans Act.

As a report to Congress states: "It is the view of the Administration that since home health agencies do not require large initial capital investments and since the growth in supply of home health services was established without any special federal grants, the grant programs should be eliminated" (DHEW, 1979).

To add to the inequity, hospitals and nursing homes had been developed and were functioning long before Medicare but there was no entity in existence that looked like a home health agency. The changes to acquire certification as a home health agency required hiring or contracting for expensive caregivers for an unknown market demand: physical, occupational, and speech therapists, medical social workers, and nurses educated in public health nursing. The new accounting procedures required sophisticated bookkeeping and planning. No new beds were needed but the development required was costly and risky and was expected to be carried out without the financial assistance or insurance given to other providers under Medicare. This led, predictably, to the growth of public home health agencies, of proprietaries, and particularly of hospital-based agencies. Voluntary agencies without public funding experienced a decrease in number; since they had been the most numerous before Medicare, the total number of home care agencies declined after the implementation of the law. Many smaller ones went out of business because they could not develop the service scope and complexity required. The proprietary agencies did grow but not as much as hospital-based ones. Proprietaries are limited in participation under Medicare because they must be licensed by the state in order to be certified for reimbursement; voluntary agencies do not have to be licensed for participation. Some states do not license any home health agencies and 21 that do have licensure laws still choose not to approve the proprietaries.

Initially this licensure requirement was meant to limit overdevelopment of proprietary agencies that could be encouraged by the favorable cost reimbursement regulations (full cost reimbursement based on ''reasonable'' costs). Without this statutory limitation, for-profit agencies could have flourished simply because of the potential for economic gain. Indeed, where proprietaries are licensed, they have 30 percent more visits and 30 percent higher costs than for comparable populations cared for by voluntary agencies (DHEW, 1979). Some proprietary agencies, for economic reasons, developed to deliver services only to patients covered by Medicare and these are now excluded from Medicare reimbursement by law (P.L. 95-142).

THE AMENDMENTS

As noted earlier, the Medicare act has been amended every year or two, primarily to increase the funding base as the program continued to cost more than had been expected, and to build in quality control and decrease fraud and abuse. Congress originally declared its intent that the federal government not become involved in the practice of medicine. However, it soon became obvious that to buy medical care with any accountability at all to the payers of that care (the public), the government had to become involved. Congress therefore adopted amendments to require quality, efficiency, and appropriateness of care and to provide sanctions against fraud and abuse. The government thus went on record that it demanded fair and appropriate service for the public dollar. Other amendments were aimed at changing eligibility to promote use of the least costly services. The amendments include these highlights:

In 1966 the initial enrollment period deadline was extended two months. The wage base for Social Security deductions was increased from $4,800 to $6,600.

In 1967 more days of inpatient care were added, durable medical equipment was covered, and the wage base for Social Security deductions was raised from $6,600 to $7,800.

In 1968 the number of inpatient days was increased again and itemized bills were required.

In 1969 cost-plus reimbursement was replaced by straight cost reimbursement.

In 1971 limits were placed on "reasonable" costs, requiring comparison with other purchasers.

In 1972 numerous substantial changes were made, including liberalization of many benefits:

- Disabled individuals were given Medicare eligibility.
- The Social Security wage base was raised to $9,000.
- Allowable expenses incurred in the last three months of the previous year could be used toward the current year's deductible.
- Allowable care in skilled nursing facilities (SNFs) was broadened to include that supervised by professional nurses.
- The copayment for Part B home health services was eliminated.

The professional standards review organization (PSRO) program, one of the most important Medicare entities, was established. This not only further defined the services Medicare would pay for but, even more importantly, it equated payment with criteria and standards of quality and appropriateness of care. PSROs focused initially on hospitals, with home health agencies included later. Cost containment was a major reason for the PSRO program, as it was for two other sections of the 1972 amendments that (1) authorized experiments and demonstration projects for prospective reimbursement trials and (2) directed that payment for any home health services be denied when prescribed by any physician found to have been habitually issuing "erroneous or inappropriate" orders for such care.

Legislative concerns for cost and quality in health care were apparent in other than Title XVIII changes in 1972. Section 1122 of the Social Security Act, certificate of need, was adopted to restrain unnecessary capital expenditures. This section authorizes denial of reimbursement for federally financed health services for the provider portion of the cost of unapproved capital expenditures and provides economic sanctions for inflationary and unneeded construction. The main target was hospital construction but home health agencies were included.

In 1973 the scope of inpatient dental services was broadened. The Social Security wage base was increased to $10,800 with provisions for it to reach $15,300 by 1976.

In 1974 the significant legislation was P.L. 93-641, the National Health Planning and Resources Development Act, not a Title XVIII amendment but Title XV of the Public Health Act, which is very influential in the delivery of home health services. This was a direct result of 1972 data on Medicare overinvestment and inflation (Hanley, 1977) and although the mandated certificate of need did not apply to home health agencies, states now could include them if they wished to do so. P.L. 93-641 set up state and regional agencies to approve applications for new services (including the capital expenditures covered under Sec. 1122) by certifying the regional need for them and the law provided direction to measure the need of existing services at a later time.

The act also allows revocation of an operating license if a provider does not comply with the certificate-of-need process for new services. The mandated certificate of need did not apply to home health agencies but this legislation permitted them to do so. Many did so choose. By 1976, 14 states included home health agencies in the CON process (Vladeck, 1980). There was opposition by health economists to this process being applied to home health agencies because it tended to limit expansion or establishment of the new services most helpful in achieving hospital cost containment and, in fact, any new service was less likely to be seen as needed than any existing one. In 1976 HEW issued a regulation removing home health agencies from CON legislation (DHEW Report, April 1979).

In 1975 waivers for nurse staffing in rural hospitals and an increase in Part B premiums were approved.

In 1976 physician fee reimbursements were protected in two minor amendments. Customary charges were protected at a higher level.

Another important year was 1977. P.L. 95-142, the Medicare-Medicaid Antifraud and Abuse Amendments, sharpened the focus on those problems. Federal audits had identified overuse, improper and unnecessary use, falsification of claims, and improper relationships (ownership of provider agencies, provider personnel assigned to agencies to increase referrals, etc.) in hospitals, skilled nursing facilities, and home health agencies. Fraud and abuse in the latter included these (Hanley, 1977):

- claims for care that did not meet conditions of participation in terms of need for skilled care
- agencies that accepted only Medicare clients, thus receiving reimbursement based on costs that were excessive and inflationary

- claims for care that was not needed or for care not given
- home health agency personnel assigned to an inpatient facility to increase referrals to that agency inappropriately
- inadequate recordkeeping, particularly by small nonprofit agencies that did not have to meet stringent audits by the Internal Revenue Service.

The other major measure that year was P.L. 95-210, the Rural Health Clinics Services Act, which increased the Social Security wage base to $16,500. It also provided for reimbursement for nurse practitioner and physician's assistant primary care in rural health clinics. The act authorized home health services for clients of those clinics by the clinic staff—a radical departure from the previous statute that mandated home care through certified home health agencies. Another standard-setting change allowed reimbursement (in rural areas only) for home care services "established" not only by a physician, but now also by nurse practitioners.

The amendments better defined the role and function of intermediaries (requiring them to provide "efficient and effective service") to include appropriate claims-processing decisions and assistance to providers to help them deliver only needed care, and authorized HEW to reassign providers where intermediaries were not doing the job. The amendments also required uniform cost reporting for all providers as well as complete disclosure of owner-provider background, and provider records, and stiffened penalties for fraud and abuse. The legislation also provided for incentive reimbursement demonstration projects.

In 1978 end stage renal disease (ESRD) patients came under Title XVIII, with special incentives for home dialysis treatment.

In 1980 the amendments, included as part of the Omnibus Reconciliation Act (P.L. 96-499), went a long way toward reducing barriers to the use of home health services: limits on the number of visits in Parts A and B were deleted; the three-day prior hospitalization requirement for Part A home health services was eliminated; states without licensure laws now could certify for-profit home health agencies for Medicare; and the Part B deductible was eliminated.

The reasons for these changes were primarily economic. Data show that few patients exceed the number of visits under Parts A and B. Those who do so have that care paid for through other federal funding so there is no public saving (HCFA Review, Winter 1981). The three-day prior hospitalization may have been costly, resulting in unnecessary expensive hospitalization in order to qualify for the home care benefit.

The objective of the 1980 amendments was to make home care more attractive, either in lieu of hospitalization or as a means of shortening the hospital stay. In localities where voluntary home health agencies were not providing adequate services, convalescent hospital stays were prolonged; for-profit agencies were given wider participation in Medicare in the hope that they would fill the service voids.

The Reconciliation Act of 1982 provided for a prospective reimbursement program for hospitalized Medicare patients. The DRG system of classifying patients and projecting average hospitalization costs was adopted in the regulations. The 8.5 percent additional payment to hospitals for nursing care of Medicare beneficiaries was deleted. Home health agency reimbursement by Medicare was set at a single cost limit for freestanding and hospital based agencies.

The amendments in the 17 years following passage of Title XVIII reflected a continuing Congressional concern for increased access, cost containment, quality, and appropriateness of services but the overwhelming focus became cost control.

THE REGULATIONS

The Medicare statute mandates that it be implemented through regulations established by HEW (now HHS). These regulations cover reimbursement methods, including definitions of "reasonable cost," "customary and prevailing charges," and many many other financial sections. Three key aims of the initial regulations formulated in 1966 are clear throughout:

1. "The intent is to reimburse *actual* costs even as they vary from institution to institution" (CFR 405.451) (emphasis added).
2. The variety of cost-finding and cost-apportionment methods all are aimed at paying for costs incurred only by the Medicare beneficiaries.
3. Payment mechanisms originally clearly favored providers but the regulations now are aimed increasingly at cost containment, even if detrimental to providers. These constraints include cost caps on services, elimination of cost-plus reimbursement, and more stringent eligibility criteria.

CFR 405.451 also states that Medicare will pay "the lesser of the reasonable cost to the beneficiary and customary charges to the general public." This caused consternation and policy revisions in nonprofit home health agencies that had subsidized traditional "free" care, or fee determined on needy clients' "ability to pay." The regulation allows Medicare to pay that reduced fee (or no fee) for its beneficiaries as the lesser of those costs. Home health agencies then face unsatisfactory alternatives: either charge everyone the full fee, effectively discouraging those who cannot pay (even if the agency were willing to accept them as bad debts), or use the annual subsidy in public/voluntary agencies as "grants" for care to certain clients. One agency that tried this felt it was establishing a "God Committee" since it no longer could provide reduced fee services.

HEW (HHS) also is authorized to put an upper limit on allowable costs based on type of service, geographical area, size of institutions, and nature and mix of services. In 1979 it put an upper limit on home health agency Medicare payments based on urban/rural location, regional labor costs, and hospital or community base. These caps no longer covered "reasonable cost" reimbursement.

'Reasonable,' 'Customary,' and 'Prevailing' Charges

Reasonable cost (used for institutional and home health services) was defined in the regulations as the full cost and the "intent is to reimburse actual costs even as they vary from institution to institution" (CFR 405.451). This encouraged the highest cost care available since it guaranteed full reimbursement.

Customary and prevailing charges are those claimed by physicians. (They are not cost based.) A customary charge is one charged the majority of clients by a professional; a prevailing charge is the one that would cover 75 percent of the customary charges in that locale. Obviously, providers who worked in a "locale" of high-priced professionals also could be reimbursed at a higher fee. This regulation not only was biased toward maldistribution of medical care but actually encouraged that kind of decreased availability.

The regulations allowed reimbursement for the lesser of the customary and prevailing charge; therefore, physicians could set their fees according to the going rate in their locale and in fact could choose a locale that allowed the highest charges and thus the highest reimbursement.

Reasonable charges and payment in full became usual in many commercial contracts following the start of Medicare. Full-cost reimbursement enhanced the idea that a fee determined by the market was valid. This whole inflationary matrix, again, was simply an incentive for physicians to choose to participate in the care of Medicare beneficiaries. It worked as long as Medicare beneficiaries lived in higher cost areas; there were no incentives for physicians to serve low-cost or low-income areas.

Another regulation that has served to limit service capacity rather than to promote growth of needed services states in part that "patients are accepted for treatment on the basis of a reasonable expectation that the patient's medical, nursing, and social needs can be met adequately by the agency in the patient's place of residence" (CFR 405.1223). This is intended to guard against unnecessary or overutilization of services. However, it implies that home health agencies have no responsibility to identify needs or to provide new or additional services but only to use existing ones appropriately.

The Role of States

Because Medicare is completely federally financed, the states have little to say regarding eligibility, payment (except for urban/rural and labor cost differences), and scope of services. States do, however, influence the delivery of services to

Medicare clients through the development of their own operating regulations. For instance, the Medicare statute specifically leaves it to the states to determine licensure of proprietary and nonprofit home health agencies. This effectively limits access to home health services, for if the state chooses not to license proprietaries, those agencies cannot qualify for Medicare. State legislation has made grants available to existing home health agencies to develop home care services for coverage seven days a week and to increase the number of services offered. These state grant funds increase the availability of home health services to Medicare's eligible population.

All parts of Medicare law—the original statute, the amendments, and the regulations—have served to limit care to those in need of medically recuperative services. The law also has been concerned with fraud and abuse, primarily through developing sanctions such as retroactive denial of payment, nonlicensure of for-profit agencies, removal of participation privilege for professionals shown to have misused Medicare payment, and monetary loss to agencies that have a pattern of providing ineligible care. Medicare issues a waiver to each home health agency that excuses it from payment for charges for ineligible care so long as ineligible claims remain less than 2.5 percent of all annual charges to Medicare; however, once an agency exceeds that percent in any one year, it is liable for all subsequent overcharges.

Medicare law has been less effective in promoting quality and appropriateness of care measures. (Those issues, as well as inflationary and expensive reimbursement problems, are discussed in Chapter 3.) However, unlike quality, cost containment efforts have been helped substantially by Medicare amendments. Even liberalizations in coverage have been aimed at cost savings; for instance, deleting beneficiary copayment for home health services was an effort to make home care more attractive than the most expensive hospital stay.

The first 17 years' experience with Medicare saw successful implementation of a universal health care system for the elderly and disabled and the testing of a model for national health insurance. Entitlement to ''free'' hospital care did not result in an onslaught by the sick elderly on the nation's hospitals. The program nonetheless had become very expensive and difficult to continue at the rate costs were increasing. Because hospital care was the most costly component, not only of Medicare but of all national health expenditures, ways of decreasing hospitalization or of providing cost-effective alternatives obviously would be welcome and necessary in future health policy.

REFERENCES

Hanley, E.J. Regulations of health facilities and services under Public Law 93-641, in H. Hyman (Ed.), *Health regulations*. Rockville, Md.: Aspen Systems Corporation, 1977.

HCFA Office of Financial and Actuarial Analysis. Personal communication, April 20, 1983.

Health Care Financing Review, Winter 1981.

Health Care Financing Review, Spring 1981.

Home care in New York State. Albany, N.Y.: Home Care Association of New York State, May 1979.

Home health care: Its utilization, costs, and reimbursement. New York: Health Services Agency of New York City, November 1977.

Home health services under Titles XVIII, XIX, and XX. Department of Health, Education, and Welfare, Report to Congress, April 1979.

Pegels, C. *Health care and the elderly.* Rockville, Md.: Aspen Systems, 1981.

Vladeck, B. *Unloving care.* New York: Basic Books, 1980.

Chapter 3

Medicare: Deficiencies and Problems

All three original aims of the Medicare legislation have been met. A method is in operation for paying the hospital bills of the elderly and thereby also assuring reimbursement to the hospitals. Second-class care has been largely eliminated; payment incentives made it advantageous for providers to give the poor, blacks, and the elderly the best of service. And by expanding the program beyond the physician lobbyists' desire that it cover only the needy elderly, Medicare provided a model for national health insurance.

In achieving these goals, a number of concessions to institutional providers and to physicians were made knowingly in the name of political necessity and many of the problems and difficulties in the legislation are byproducts of those compromises. The concessions created substantive deficiencies in the program. Because it was an entitlement program, broad compliance by institutional providers was absolutely necessary.

As noted earlier, a recurring nightmare for the legislative framers was that the newly entitled sick elderly would descend upon the hospitals and that they would be turned away for lack of beds or the institutions' lack of interest. Therefore, the law had to be made attractive to hospitals. Physicians, too, needed incentives to participate, including those that were only partly monetary. Other than the assurance of optimum payment, physicians also needed to know that their authority in providing medical care would be untouched by government. Because these providers were absolutely necessary for the delivery of effective Medicare services, the law gave them generous payments and a federal hands-off policy in terms of evaluating the medical care; cost and quality measures suffered greatly.

COST CONTAINMENT IGNORED

The Medicare law not only assured optimal payment to providers but made no attempt at cost containment. That concern did not begin to surface until later, in the regulations.

Reasonable cost for institutional reimbursement and repayment of customary and prevailing charges for physicians were acknowledgments that Medicare would pay full cost and the market price for services. In addition, costs were repaid at the time of reimbursement, not at the time the expenses were incurred, which made possible payment in excess of actual costs or charges. This was a radical departure from pre-1965 insurance reimbursement, which had been provided on a fixed rate or amount set prospectively. Historical data for home care costs were essentially nonexistent before Medicare so it was difficult to assess reasonableness of cost for home health services under that program.

Other incentives were offered to the insurance companies that were the claims processors for Medicare. Blue Cross received about 90 percent of the intermediary contracts under Part A and Blue Shield about 60 percent of the Part B carrier contracts (Van Dyke & Elliot, 1969). That the providers chose these insurance groups was hardly surprising—they had had a long relationship. Blue Cross was established in 1929 for the express purpose of assuring payment to hospitals.

Medicare provided the intermediaries and carriers with an economically secure and risk-free role in which they were paid in full for what they disbursed, plus administrative costs. Unlike other insurance ventures, they had no liability for disbursements over and above the funds available to pay for the benefits. There was, therefore, no incentive for the claims processors to hold down costs.

Hospitals meanwhile experienced further deficits that led to their raising prices in an attempt to meet increased costs. No standardized accounting was required so the variety of providers' cost billings increased administrative costs in claims processors' offices. The absence of standardized accounting also enabled hospitals to submit the highest possible allowable costs for reimbursement.

The Medicare law not only lacked cost containment measures, it encouraged inflationary actions.

For example, to assure that hospitals would not provide second-class care to beneficiaries, Medicare paid only for services actually delivered. The average hospital cost per diem, including for example maternity and pediatrics services, could not be used to determine the per diem amount that Medicare would reimburse. That daily reimbursable rate was determined on only the services used by Medicare patients. However, that rate tended to be the most beneficial of all to third party payers because it was a guarantee of full cost reimbursement (Feder, 1977). Hospitals saw this favorable payment process as an incentive to purchase and develop high-quality expensive services and equipment for the care of elderly patients.

The sophistication and cost of care of the elderly rose dramatically following 1965; in fact, 25 percent of all Medicare monies were spent on hospital care for elderly patients in their last 12 months of life (Ginzberg, 1977). This led to even greater medical care costs outside the Medicare population as expensive services and equipment that the program reimbursed for its beneficiaries then became available to the general public. The sophistication and cost of medical care both were increased greatly by Medicare funding.

A similar cause of overall health care cost inflation was the way Blue Cross chose to change its policies when the elderly went under Medicare coverage. Since Blue Cross premiums are experience rated, and since the highest use and highest cost group of subscribers was the elderly, premiums might be expected to drop when that expensive group was provided with other coverage. Not so. Blue Cross did not drop premiums to the level where they would cover costs, but instead used the revenues to cover new and expanded services under its policies. Insurance coverage removes the one price barrier to use of services (they appear to be free) and therefore not only were more services covered but their use also increased (Feder, 1977).

Medicare's full cost reimbursement of customary and prevailing fees served to allow and even encourage physician charges to rise, not only for Medicare patients, but for all patients (Hollahan et al., 1977). Medicare reimbursement in effect encourages physicians to practice where high fees are acceptable—usually high-income areas. In addition, physicians' participation in Medicare is voluntary and they can opt, instead, for billing patients their full self-set fee and require them to obtain the amount allowed by Medicare by submitting their own bills. Physician reimbursement for inpatients is higher than for outpatient care, thereby encouraging expensive hospitalization for Medicare beneficiaries (Hollahan et al., 1977).

EFFECTS ON HOME HEALTH SERVICES

Parts of the law specifically addressing home health services also were inflationary. The statutory requirement that patients must use expensive skilled services in order to be eligible for others, such as home health aide care causes those costly elements to be provided even when unnecessary just to achieve eligibility for other needed treatment. Although requiring skilled care was meant to limit services to acute care (instead of chronic care), skilled care requires the most expensive care givers.

The duplication and overlap of services under Titles XVIII (Medicare), XIX (Medicaid), and XX (federal-state social service programs) of the Social Security Act led to highly inflationary costs. Particularly in home care, it is possible to shift patients from one program to the other as eligibility lapses. One home health agency has documented switching a patient 28 times between different payment sources in order to continue providing service (DHEW, 1979). The dual purpose of paying for care of the elderly while also ensuring providers optimal payment to assure their participation also was inflationary.

THE QUALITY PROBLEM

Quality also has been a victim in the battle to have providers accept Medicare. Although discrimination and two-class care were reduced by the payment incentives in the statute (even early nonparticipant southern hospitals that were reluctant to desegregate found it worth their while to accept these changes), other omissions of quality are critical deficits in the Medicare law.

Vladeck, in his book on nursing home policy (1980), makes the case for quality in publicly funded health care: waste, or buying low quality with one's own money is, at worst, a foolish transfer of funds between buyer and seller but when the buying is done with someone else's money (tax dollars) and even then the service does not go to the fund provider, then quality is essential. Considering the important issue of accountability to the public for use of its funds, the omission of quality assurance in the act was a high price to pay in order to please the care providers.

Efforts to increase quality have been hampered by leaving the direction of those attempts in the hands of the providers. For instance, utilization review and professional standards review organizations are run by physicians. Even in home care, where they rarely see the patients throughout the entire episode of care, it still is the doctors who establish and review the treatment plans and certify the appropriateness of those services for Medicare.

Quality in home health care has been poorly defined and rarely monitored. Although quality can be defined many ways (e.g., patient satisfaction or effective medical outcomes) the Medicare law addresses only the access and process of care, leaving its component elements to be determined by physicians. This is apparent in the first section of the statute (Title XVIII, Sec. 1801), which states that it does not authorize "any federal officer to exercise any supervision or control over the practice of medicine or the manner in which medical services are delivered." This, known as the nonintervention clause, has been the primary roadblock to building any process or outcome measurements of Medicare.

UTILIZATION AND REVIEW

Appropriate utilization of services was considered in framing the legislation and the utilization review (UR) requirement ultimately was included. However, UR was required only for hospital care, thereby allowing (or encouraging) inappropriate Medicare service utilization in other areas. Even in hospitals, UR lacked sanctions or leverage against inappropriate care until the fraud and abuse amendments of 1977 (P.L. 95-142).

Another important reason that appropriateness of care was neglected was because of the choice of claims payment agency. As noted, the original Social

Security Act was passed to provide benefits different from those of Medicare: cash. The Social Security Administration disbursed money to those who met eligibility requirements; the quality of use of that money was never measured, only eligibility for it. The agency's personnel and policies therefore were geared to timely and accurate disbursement and it had no reason to have developed methods for assessing quality, appropriateness, or cost effectiveness of benefits.

When Medicare was passed, Congress felt that the Social Security Administration was the logical agency to administer claims payment; it had the needed bureaucracy in place and Medicare was, after all, another Social Security program. This decision sanctioned payment without quality assessment, even though Medicare benefits are services, not dollars, and therefore can be subjected to various evaluations.

Deficits other than cost, quality, and utilization are apparent in the legislation. There was the problem of access—to physicians and to home health services. Part of the physician access problem was and still is maldistribution. Not only does the act provide no incentives for appropriate distribution of existing medical personnel but the incentives it does include are for just the opposite—to offer services where reimbursement is highest and need is lowest. As for development of new, needed services or for additional basic home health agencies, the funding sources just are not there, nor are other incentives (Trager, 1971).

Two important deficiencies in the act probably were unavoidable and all center on the unpredictability of behaviors following the passage of Medicare:

1. The statute is one of entitlement. This means that everyone who meets the criteria is entitled to the benefits, both now and in the future. Although the number of over-65 individuals was known, their use of benefits was not predictable. Because of this huge margin for error, the legislative drafting focused on accommodation with providers, whose full cooperation was imperative.
2. Hospital participation had to be voluntary (if the hospital lobby was to approve passage of the act) so wide concessions and incentives to providers were necessary. Even with hospital cooperation, it was not clear whether enough beds would be available for the feared onslaught of sick elderly (as noted in Chapter 2).

COPAYMENTS AND DEDUCTIBLES

Since the Omnibus Reconciliation Bill of 1980 deleted Part B home health service deductibles, all home care under Medicare has been available without prior hospitalization, copayments, or deductibles. The economics of funding federal health programs, however, already has resulted in proposals for cost sharing by Medicare patients for their health care. Copayments and deductibles will again become a major part of the Medicare payment system, and this reintroduces a number of inequities.

Deductibles and copayments are costs to the beneficiaries and are intended to reduce overall program expenses and services. In practice, these costs determine use on the basis of individuals' wealth and not by their need. Not only are the wealthier aged better able to use the services but they tend to need them less, for many diseases of the elderly poor can be traced to inadequate diet and lack of preventive services. The regressive nature of the Social Security tax as the funding base for Part A has been criticized widely because rich and poor employees alike contribute the same amounts and these payments are far easier for those with higher incomes. When it is realized that it is the rich who can use the services more freely (they can afford the deductibles and copayments), the inequity of the system becomes more apparent.

One argument in favor of such a regressive tax, of course, is that every beneficiary has earned it equally, having contributed in an equal way; the benefits thus become ''rights.'' A second argument against such a tax-based system is that Medicare (or other Social Security benefits) are being paid for by current workers for the current aged and it therefore is a welfare system, not an earned benefit, since there is no fund of past earnings.

Individual premiums and money from general revenues fund Part B. These premiums, like copayments and deductibles, do little to reduce ultimate costs and burden poorer beneficiaries at the expense of the richer ones. This, too, is a regressive measure that tends to reduce access to care to those who need it most. The inequities in favor of the wealthier go further than the standard cost of monthly premiums. Because the wealthier also have much better access to care and a wider range of services, the poorer beneficiaries are doubly compromised on access as well as on the economic barrier of the premiums.

Davis (1975) in an assessment of equity under Medicare, finds wide disparities between different income levels. Her study shows that the higher the income of the recipients, the higher the reimbursement from Medicare; they also utilize higher quality and more specialized services. A larger percentage of enrollees in the top income brackets utilize services; the number of services per patient also rises with income. Inequities by race also are apparent, with whites proportionately using more services than blacks, especially in nursing homes. The only higher utilization by blacks is in hospital outpatient departments. Regional differences in the cost of providing and buying services also are inequitable with a standardized nationwide premium. This system again favors the rich and those where access is easy.

PROBLEMS INEVITABLE

Major problems with Medicare have been identified. As noted, cost containment, quality, and equity all were sacrificed to the political necessity of encouraging provider participation. Could these problems have been avoided by more skillful policy decisions? Hindsight is a powerful analytical tool, but even with that benefit it is hard to see how the initial legislation could have been completely devoid of such deficiencies. Perhaps reimbursement could have been less inflationary and still satisfied providers and perhaps a delay in implementation of the program would have been worthwhile in order to develop an intermediary claims processing group that, unlike the Social Security agency, would have looked at appropriateness and quality before payment.

The political clout of the organized medical community, however, was not overstated. Physicians have long used their influence effectively on self-interest legislation (Harris, 1966). In fact, national health insurance legislation was left out of the original Social Security measure for fear that the American Medical Association would defeat it (Feder, 1977).

The Medicare program, which was the first effort to offer health services on a nationwide basis, provided "equal treatment and unequal benefits" (Davis, 1975). Local application of multisite programs has been recognized as uniformly difficult (Clinton, 1979), and when equity also is required, it is even more of a problem. Equity suffered primarily because the program was an entitlement approach. Eligibility for predetermined benefits was the first priority, and only when that was assured could utilization of services be addressed.

The regulations and subsequent amendments have sought to remedy the problems in the original law and how it has come to be implemented. Much still was needed, however, before the Medicare model could be utilized for a universal national health insurance system.

REFERENCES

Clinton, C.A. *Local success and federal failure.* Cambridge, Mass.: ABT Books, 1979.

Davis, K. Equal treatment and unequal benefits: The Medicare program. *Milbank Memorial Fund Quarterly,* Fall 1975.

Feder, J. Medicare implementation and the policy process. *Journal of Health Policy, Politics & Law,* Summer 1977, *3*(2).

Ginzberg, E. *The limits of health reform.* New York: Basic Books, Inc., 1977.

Harris, R. *A sacred trust.* New York: New American Library, 1966.

Home health services under Titles XVIII, XIX, and XX. Department of Health, Education, and Welfare, Report to Congress, April 1979.

Hollahan, J., Spitz, B., Pollak, W., & Feder, J. *Altering Medicaid provider reimbursement methods.* Wash., D.C.: The Urban Institute, June 1977.

Omnibus Reconciliation Act of 1980 (includes Medicare amendments on reimbursement to contractors and elimination of home health service deductibles in Part B).

P.L. 89-97, Social Security Amendments of 1965 (Medicare, Medicaid).

Social Security Act Amendments of 1975 (Federal-State Social Service Programs).

P.L. 95-142, Fraud and Abuse Amendments to the SSA, 1977.

Trager, B. Home health services and health insurance. *Medical Care,* January-Feburary 1971.

Van Dyke, F. & Elliot, R. *Military Medicare.* Wash., D.C.: U.S. Dept. of Defense, 1969.

Vladek, B. *Unloving care.* New York: Basic Books, Inc., 1980.

Chapter 4

Home Health Services and the Medicare Influence

Home health services today are a product of public policy. Medicare has shaped them into a medical framework. This has overshadowed the historical mission of home care, which over the years had been more concerned with support, assistance, and nursing care. Whether this shift in emphasis and structure is good or bad depends on whether the objective is economy, social welfare, or increased health status. How this change in focus came about can be understood best by looking at the original goals in the making of home care policy and at the cultural background in which those decisions were made.

Care of health in communities became an important endeavor in the last half of the 19th century in America. Industrialization, increased mobility through the opening of railroads, and the rise of urban life produced many efforts in support of public health ventures. State and local boards of health were formed, disease prevention was beginning to be understood, and nursing was a growing profession. This last aspect of public health development is important, since nurses always have been involved in the delivery of home care services.

THE BEGINNINGS: LILLIAN WALD

The first organized home nursing service was established in 1893 by Lillian Wald as the Visiting Nurse Service of New York City, as part of the Henry Street Settlement services to the city's poor. By 1909 she had persuaded the Metropolitan Life Insurance Company to begin a home nursing service for its policyholders in New York City. The pilot project was so successful it was adopted in many other communities by other insurance companies by the 1920s. The carriers paid the full cost of the home services offered (Leahy, Cobb, & Jones, 1972).

The nursing profession continued to flourish in the 20th century, with home care as a continued component. By 1900, 20 agencies similar to the Visiting Nurse Service had been established to serve the urban poor. In 1910, Teachers College of Columbia University instituted the first graduate program for community health nurses. The National Organization for Public Health Nursing was established in 1912.

The same year home care for rural communities was pioneered as a visiting nurse service through the Red Cross. The nurses worked independently in these communities, providing service to the sick, well-baby care, and school nursing. County health departments began adopting this plan, nearly all of them employing nurses to provide home care in rural areas. As automobiles became common, the visiting nurse services grew. Public health nursing became part of the Yale School of Nursing's basic curriculum in 1923 and by the end of World War II was part of all collegiate preparation in nursing.

During World War II physicians began limiting their practice to their offices and to hospitals, rather than making home visits; there was a shortage of physicians during the war and they could be far more efficient if patients went to them. A pragmatic point was that they also could make more money if they saw more patients. As a result of this change, visiting nurse associations grew rapidly to fill the need for care in the home. In 1946 Montefiore Hospital in New York City developed a team approach for posthospital acute care and the idea for convalescent home care was born. During this same time the first paraprofessional home services—homemakers—became available for a fee.

Because home care services in the United States began as a professional nursing endeavor, their evolution followed a route different from that in Europe. Such services there generally began as part of Europe's version of the social security system and therefore were a governmentally subsidized entitlement. Because of the broad constituency, the services tended to be those that were not costly and could be available to everyone relatively inexpensively.

This led to the initial use of "home helps" rather than professional nurses for the care delivery. Home helps are what are known in the United States as home health aides and homemakers. These paraprofessionals generally are trained with public funds and are made available through public community-based service networks. Communities receive these services as part of their health care entitlement.

The great majority of persons using these services are the elderly and the disabled; for example, in England, 88 percent of those receiving care from home helps are over 65. The proportion of paraprofessionals to population is four times greater in England than in the United States (DHEW, April 1979). This is a reflection of the difference in perspective on the kinds of care to be governmentally provided.

THE MEDICAL-BASED MODEL

The age of the Social Security system in the United States is not the only reason for the different emphasis. Two other cultural factors in this country have influenced the home care framework:

1. There is more emphasis here on personal responsibility in family structure and less likelihood that governmentally financed health care would substitute for services usually provided by relatives.
2. The institutional approach to health care is much stronger and better established in the United States, as is the appreciation of efficiency in all areas (DHEW, April 1979).

It is not surprising, therefore, that home care services in this country tended more toward the medical model and were provided by professionals.

Home help paraprofessional groups did not appear on the American health care scene until midway through the 20th century. Homemakers were the first, often were financed by welfare funds for the poor, and were available through some visiting nurse agencies. Home health aides as a group were defined first in the Kerr-Mills Medical Assistance for the Aged (MAA) act in 1960. They were defined as health caregivers (similar to hospital aides) and thus considered separate from homemakers.

Although MAA was poorly received and very few states chose to participate in the program, Medicaid five years later was built on many of its strengths. What survived well was the concept of home health aides. In 1961 the Community Health Services and Facilities Act was passed to develop noninstitutional services. Funds were made available for training home health aides and for adding them to existing programs, especially home care in rural areas.

Before Medicare, most home care was being delivered by Voluntary Visiting Nurse Agencies, with few proprietaries providing service (there was no profit in it) and with few public agencies providing it except in rural areas. Nursing was the main service offered, with some homemaker and home health aide availability.

Most of the care delivered was to the elderly who suffered from chronic conditions and who needed subacute nursing care. A typical visit included bathing the patient, reviewing self-care (nutrition, elimination), and attending to such tasks as vitamin or insulin injections or dressings for chronic ulcers. Payment was either through welfare agencies or privately on a sliding scale of fees subsidized by charitable organizations such as churches or the Community Chest type of entity.

Medicare changed not only the payment source but also the eligibility of patients, the agency delivery system, and the purpose of care given. Medicare covered home care under both Parts A and B. The purpose was to substitute home care for extended and costlier hospitalization. Because it was to fulfill only this narrow need, eligibility was determined on the basis of the acute care condition: whether the patient was homebound, needed skilled care, and was under a physician's treatment plan. Even the homebound condition had to arise from the medical basis.

Skilled care means medically directed service given by a nurse or other professional therapist and aimed only at convalescence from an episode of illness. In addition, this care must be planned, reviewed, and certified as necessary by the referring physician. Before the federal government began paying health bills, it was not seen as necessary or even appropriate for physicians to direct home care. Ever since the first Henry Street Settlement services were established more than 70 years before Medicare, nurses had independently and safely delivered home care to the sick, the disabled, and children.

PHYSICIANS AND HOME HEALTH CARE

There were reasons for requiring physician direction and certification of need in Medicare home health services, however:

- Medicare (even the home health services) was limited to medical treatment, not maintenance or support services or care for chronic conditions. Medical care means medical direction.
- An overwhelming concern in all of the Medicare entitlement process was that services might not be available for every beneficiary who might claim eligibility.

Therefore, to assure that there would be some way to limit services to those who were truly in need of them, the system required some kind of gatekeeper. The only persons Congress regarded as gatekeepers to health services were physicians. It also was politically necessary to keep assuring physicians that Medicare would not intrude on their traditional direction of health care—even to the point of adding physician direction to the historically nonmedical home care services.

Unfortunately, most physicians did not seem to understand or value home care, and few of those practicing in 1965 had ever made a house call or knew what kind of health service was needed in the home. A physician writing in a medical journal stated: ''Because community health problems are essentially medical, the medical profession should maintain the leadership in the provision of those services'' (Taubenhaus, 1965). He prophesied that the focus of community medicine would remain on the eradication of disease, missing the point entirely on prevention of disease and health maintenance. He added that care of the elderly would increasingly require costly medical specialists, again missing the larger problem of chronic care and nonacute disabilities. His view on home care was that it would "aid in keeping the patient in the community where the traditional physician-patient relationship may be maintained."

Taubenhaus was not alone in his views of the specialized medical nature of care needed by the elderly. An editorial in *The New York Times* on the day Medicare went into effect, July 1, 1966, said the ultimate answer to care of the elderly "lies in more medical schools, more hospitals and a big expansion in Extended Care Facilities." It was mistakenly believed the elderly would need more highly acute care, whereas their needs are for more support services. Home care was viewed by those formulating Medicare coverage as an extension of medically directed acute care (Senate hearings, 1964). There was no awareness that care needed in the home, even if it were simply part of a medical spectrum, might require some of the same maintenance assistance supplied in the hospital such as meals, laundry, and a safe environment. Somehow if patients were able to go home from the hospital, they therefore must be able to fulfill all their needs other than the intermittent skilled care services. Of course, they also had to be homebound, but not so much so that they could not take care of themselves. (Without the homebound status, patients could go to their physicians' offices, so it remained as a home care criterion.)

Homemakers vs. Home Health Aides

When the first Medicare bill went to Congress in 1961 it provided coverage for homemakers in the home care benefits. The bill failed, mainly because it did not assure physician autonomy. The revised bill, submitted in 1964, met the physician concerns and deleted homemakers from home care benefits, replacing them with home health aide services. This change reflected the same distinction that Kerr-Mills MAA legislation had made: homemakers were a welfare benefit, home health aides a health benefit. The change also was a subtle reflection of an overwhelming focus in Medicare: that it was a medical benefit for sickness care, not a maintenance program for the disabled elderly.

In regard to home care the *Medicare Manual* states: "The aged person who is feeble and insecure (without a medical condition causing it) doesn't qualify" (Chapter 2, Part 208.4). This perspective has greatly limited home care eligibility: not only must Medicare enrollees need to present an acute illness or injury requiring home care service, they also must need professional skilled nursing care.

The Dramatic Change and Its Effect on Costs

Actuarial experts testifying in the 1961 hearings on the first Medicare bill (Senate, 1964) had estimated that home care costs would not be increased significantly, partly because the service capacity did not exist and partly because savings in decreased hospital care would nearly make up for the difference in increased use of home services. Another actuarial witness had estimated that $1 per beneficiary per year would cover the Part B nonhospital home health benefits. Obviously, events proved the experts wrong.

Medicare obviously changed the home care system dramatically. No longer directed and provided by nurses for patients' long-term needs, home service now is a medical adjunct to acute care, and for all their lack of skill and interest in this care, it is physicians who are nominally directing the system. This has added immeasurably to the cost of care.

Although home care expenditures, even at their highest, were 2.6 percent of all Medicare payments, they were far costlier than had been predicted. This is partly because of their use in addition to hospitalization rather than in substitution, partly because Medicare reimbursement practices increased health care cost inflation, and partly because of the rise in overall health expenditures. Another high cost factor can be traced to the eligibility criteria that require each beneficiary to utilize expensive skilled services before any other allowed services or supplies can be made available.

Physicians, as do most professionals, tend to implement the therapies that they know best, value, and use in their own work. Therefore, home care, traditionally a low-technology and low-cost venture, under Medicare has become a service filled with high-cost care. It is not unusual for a physician to order a battery of expensive blood tests rather than make a home visit, or to utilize physical therapists for routine range of motion or ambulation of homebound patients. Physicians should be aware that nurses can teach families to carry out these exercises or that a visiting nurse's assessment and history can tell more than blood tests in many cases.

Impact on the Marketplace for Home Care

This new medical focus also changed the marketplace for home care services. It became very difficult for the nonindigent elderly to get moderate cost maintenance care in the home. This resulted from the underlying assumption in the Medicare law that if care was "really needed," meaning related to a medical episode, then Medicare would cover it. If Medicare would not cover it, this view held, then the individuals should pay from their own pockets for such a "luxury."

The "luxury" of patient maintenance at home once was affordable on a self-care basis, since the agencies providing that kind of service were fairly uncomplicated, with little overhead, paperwork, or expensive services other than nursing. Home health agencies now are big business, with sophisticated recordkeeping, mandated committee and utilization review work, and a range of expensive skilled professionals on payroll. Maintenance care from such an agency costs a lot of money.

Even though Medicare policy restricted use of home care, it led to increased availability and access to services in other ways. In 1963 there were 1,163 agencies in the United States offering home nursing service but in 1966 fewer than 250 of them had the range of services to meet the Medicare criteria for a home health agency. During the first decade of Medicare, those that met home health agency standards increased by 71 percent to about 430. The most growth was in hospital-based agencies. There also was some increase in proprietaries, from a very small number to 15 percent of all home health agencies by 1979, when there was a total of 3,000 (DHEW, April 1979).

The mainstay of pre-Medicare home care agencies, the voluntary Visiting Nurse agencies, decreased after 1965 because it was too expensive and risky for small entities to build the care components needed for Medicare eligibility. It was difficult for home health agencies to survive the lack of stable funding (most federal monies for noninstitutional care development predated Medicare), and the uncertain and changing reimbursement policy.

Patients in institutions (hospitals and nursing homes) essentially are full-service clients and their care is reimbursed on a per diem rate based on use of existing resources. Home care patients, however, do not use full services in every instance and the agency is reimbursed only for those utilized. For instance, if home health aides hired by an agency are not used 100 percent, the reimbursement for their services may be less than their cost. This means the agency may suffer financially from the uncertain demand on its services, a financial risk that is somewhat less of a problem for institutions. Agencies that had initially added services to be Medicare eligible found that their reimbursement was not sufficient to cover those extra services' costs, so they dropped their Medicare eligibility. In this way the number of agencies decreased and the average size of agencies grew.

Certificate-of-need legislation (CON) was passed as part of P.L. 93-641, the Health Planning and Resources Development Act of 1974, to restrict the growth of unnecessary health services. It was mandated for institutions but home health agencies could be included by states' options. Fourteen states chose to do so. That also has limited availability of service since the need for a new service is often harder to justify than adding capability to existing services.

STATUS OF HOME HEALTH SERVICES

The availability of home health services has increased in both urban and rural areas but to a considerably lesser degree in the latter. Home health agencies provide direct nursing care but, unlike the proprietaries, can contract out for other needs, including physical, speech, and occupational therapy; medical social services; and home health aides. These usually are contracted from other agencies or institutions because such ancillary services are less in demand and a fee-for-service basis is more economical than hiring caregivers on a full-time basis. Such contracting is easy in urban areas but the services are not readily available in rural areas so entities there cannot easily obtain and/or provide the minimal service components to qualify as home health agencies.

This obviously leads to a great disparity between urban and rural access to home health services: 90 percent of Medicare beneficiaries in urban areas have availability as compared with only 55 percent of those in rural areas. Utilization rates are similar: 3 percent of urban beneficiaries use home health services as compared with 1.5 percent in rural areas (DHEW, April 1979). Another factor in uncertain availability has been the way funds under Title XX of the Social Security Act have been expended. This section authorizes transfer of federal funds to states as grants-in-aid to develop and provide a variety of social services for the elderly. Home health services may be included and states may or may not decide to use the funds for them. Often the very areas most in need of such services also are most lacking a variety of other social assistance such as nutrition programs and, especially in rural areas, transportation to health care centers. Therefore, while Title XX could be used to meet home health needs, that may not be the first priority.

Medicare has increased access to home health services for the elderly, at least for their acute care convalescence needs. No deductible or copayment is required. As noted in earlier chapters, prior hospitalization no longer is required, the skilled care criterion has been somewhat liberalized to allow for teaching and counseling in certain circumstances, and the homebound criterion allows patients to make trips away from the home for medical care.

However, access for nonmedical home health services has been made more difficult. Reasonable cost reimbursement allows full repayment for the highest quality care. This induces agencies to develop and offer high-quality high-cost services, and for those who need care not covered by Medicare (e.g., maintenance and prevention services), the expense is prohibitive.

HOSPITAL-BASED HOME CARE AND NURSING HOMES

Medicare home health services were meant to substitute for hospitalization or nursing home placement. About 80 percent of home care patients are posthospital referrals (HCFA, 1980). The others are referred by physicians after an outpatient episode of illness or by family or friends when they are unable to manage for themselves following an illness. When patients who have been sent home for care become too dependent or too ill to be cared for there, nearly all return to the hospital instead of going directly to a nursing home.

A number of factors account for the strong home care-hospital relationship and the almost total absence (2 percent) of referrals to nursing homes from home care. Both hospital treatment and Medicare home service require skilled caregivers, with the medical acuteness of the case determining where care is delivered. Medicare covers about 75 percent of all home care patients and Medicaid 60 percent of those in nursing homes (Fox & Clauser, 1980). Medicare requires skilled services and a short-term recuperative process. Rarely can this requirement be met by nursing home residents, so Medicare patients who develop longer term maintenance requirements usually have to gain Medicaid eligibility or pay privately for nursing home care. Conversely, nursing home residents who generally have been receiving supportive care, must need skilled acute care in order to be accepted under Medicare home health services.

Medicaid covers home health care in some states as an optional benefit (it is required under Medicare), as noted earlier in this chapter. Although most states have opted to cover home care under their Medicaid programs, most also have chosen to cover only welfare recipients under Medicaid and not provide more liberalized benefits for the medically indigent as well.

The Isolation Factor

Other than the different constituencies in the two levels of care, and the different kinds of services needed, an important factor is that the majority of nursing home residents have no family members and nearly two-thirds of home care patients live with other family members (DHEW, Nov. 1979). This isolation factor makes a difference in where given patients will obtain care and whether they are likely to transfer to or from a nursing home. Patients who have family assistance are more likely to be maintained at home, even when they have the same level of disability as the majority of nursing home residents; a nursing home is the care setting of last resort.

It has been estimated that between 25 percent and 50 percent of nursing home residents could be maintained on home care by the addition of some maintenance services such as assistance with meal preparation, laundry, and shopping (Vladeck, 1980; Hammond, 1979). These services are not available now in home care because there is no reimbursement for them. Consequently, many patients end up in nursing homes simply for the lack of support services. Only those needing 24-hour care would be in nursing homes if intermittent self-care needs could be provided in the community. Vladeck (1980) suggests that 40 percent of nursing home days are used by chronically ill isolated patients who could be cared for in the community for the same amount of money. That would be half a million individuals.

Home health services have not been developed to meet the maintenance and support needs of patients, and the reimbursement potential is not there either. Since the vast majority (80 percent) of home health care is now paid for with public dollars, government can effectively define what the marketplace will offer. Underdevelopment of maintenance services therefore reflects the absence of a public payment program for such care. Even when services are reimbursable, their development is limited by policy in order to limit public expenditures. Legislators have been loathe to increase individuals' eligibility without adequate service capacity, and agencies, worrying about adequate reimbursement, are reluctant to increase capacity without assurance it will be used and paid for.

Increasing capacity and eligibility are far riskier for government in home care services than in institutional care. If construction of facilities or beds is limited, so, too, is service availability. In home health services, however, once an agency has developed the services and administrative mechanisms to satisfy Medicare requirements for participation, all that is needed to increase services is additional personnel—professional, paraprofessional, and nonprofessional. This can be accomplished relatively easily, so service outlays (and public expenditures) then can double in a very short time. In home care, the most effective way of controlling costs is to limit eligibility for services. Costs per home care visit have risen just as rapidly as other fees per service but the number of home visits has remained low. Home service costs account for only 2.6 percent of all Medicare expenditures and for only 12 percent of all public spending for long-term care.

Changes in Legislative Priorities

Federal underdevelopment of home services also can be traced to the rapid change in legislative priorities in health care funding that leaves inadequate time for the development of programs before Congress turns to new concepts or approaches. In 1961, Congress voted $42 million for the development of home health services over a six-year period (Milio, 1975). In 1965 it added $9 million because of the home care entitlements under Medicare and Medicaid. In the next 15 years interest grew (and funding followed) for noninstitutional services other than home care. In 1970 federal funding priorities switched to regionalizing specialty medical services, in 1972 the focus turned to ambulatory care, in 1973 the goal became primary care, and from 1974 through 1977 the chief beneficiaries were health maintenance organizations and rural health (Milio, 1975). Funding for home health services dropped dramatically from 1968 to 1975, and in 1980 the federal budget contained no allotment whatsoever for their development. By 1983 there was increased interest in the costs saving aspects of home care, and funds were provided for the establishment of home health agencies in low-use areas.

Legislative advocacy for home health services is weak for several reasons:

- The primary constituents are old and without energy or ability to demand legislative action; the children of the very old are their main caregivers, and most of them also tend to be old.
- Physicians have no monetary gain or interest in home care, and nurses involved in home care are a tiny minority of the profession.

- Both Congressional committees on the aging lack the authority to send bills directly to the floor and must wait for a broader acceptance of the issues before action can be taken (Sager, 1979).
- Congress feared that if the federal government began to pay for supportive home care, families that had been providing those services free would stop doing so and rely on government funds instead (Bellin, 1972). This last could prove to be a huge expense and was not viewed by Congress as a true health benefit since it is not part of medical care, but is seen as a key to the U.S. Treasury for homemaker services.

At the time of Medicare's passage, home care was primarily a supportive nursing service. There were no good records of its cost and there was great confusion about its aims. With so little known about past home health services it was very difficult to plan with any assurance for the future or to know how to measure their usefulness.

Clearly the intent of Medicare home health services was to focus on medical convalescence, not supportive nursing care, and limitations were developed to assure federal payment of only those medically needed. What was missing were incentives to encourage the use of home health services instead of institutionalization. There are no incentives for physicians to refer patients to home health agencies; the more patients doctors have in a hospital, the more efficient and the more profitable it is to care for them there.

In addition, physicians understand acute care and need only plan for the medical services needed for patients, who already are supplied with the hotel services in a hospital (laundry, meals, heat, bedclothes, safety). The doctors can feel secure that they are doing a good job (and are being reimbursed well for it) so why refer patients to another agency for convalescent care? Physicians may have little knowledge of what is going on in the home yet are held responsible for ordering and reviewing the care given there—with no reimbursement for doing so.

To add to the problem, home care, especially of the elderly, is not very interesting to physicians. They tend to prefer to treat the elderly in a medical episodic way in the office or the hospital and cease their intervention (and responsibility) if the patients are not acutely ill. The lack of physicians' incentives for home care use is critical for it is they who are gatekeepers to the services; without their interest, acquiescence and, at the very least, their referral and orders, patients cannot receive Medicare-reimbursed home care services.

Incentives for Hospitals Lacking

Similarly, there are few incentives for hospitals to encourage the use of home health services. Hospitals are reimbursed at full cost for the administrative functions in referring patients to home care. Considering the economic benefits in full cost reimbursement, there may be a small profit in such administrative efforts. Inappropriate hospitalization can result in retroactive denial of payment for the nonacute care days provided, but hospitals can send patients home more easily when they can accomplish the home care referrals.

There is no good reason for hospitals to use home health services in lieu of inpatient care if it can be shown that an individual still is eligible to be treated as an inpatient. If they lacked beds, hospitals would have an economic (and social) reason for moving patients out as soon as possible but there are few shortages and empty beds are not profitable. The major source of referrals—hospitals and, ultimately, physicians—therefore have no vested interest in using or encouraging home care for their patients. This has been a primary reason for the low utilization and underdevelopment of those services.

A number of administrative problems affect Medicare home health services. Foremost is cost. Home health services are supposed to substitute for institutionalization and therefore save money; however, studies show that they are primarily add-ons (Hammond, 1979; Weissert, 1980). Hospital length of stay has decreased under Medicare but there is little evidence that home care is one of the causes or that it is used in lieu of extended institutionalization. The decrease in length of stay probably is a result of regulation (primarily utilization review activities mandated by Medicare and adopted by insurance companies) but the increased number and technological intensity of services have cancelled out any cost savings from shorter stays.

Patients who use homemakers and other supportive home services have lower mortality and higher use of other services, including hospitalization (Weissert, 1980). Berkman and Syme (1979) show that strong social networks for the elderly in their community also lead to decreased mortality. These findings indicate that maintaining the elderly in their communities, with support services, will prolong their lives. The costs of increased longevity of the disabled and ill elderly are a moral dilemma in health care policy.

Ethics vs. Economics in Policymaking

Unlike traditional measurement of the cost-effectiveness of medical care that increases the life and therefore the productivity of nonelderly patients, prolonging the life of the nonproductive elderly is a cost that must be weighed against other potential health care benefits that could be achieved with those same dollars. It is an ethical as well as an economic question and one that must be asked, and answered, in the making of health policy. Essentially the investment of spending dollars on care of the elderly will lead to even greater costs, not less.

The answer does not rest simply on investment in economic productivity or on health vs. social costs or on family vs. governmental responsibility, but it does involve all three of those issues. The outcome desired will have a lot to do with cost-effectiveness measurement so the traditional economic productivity equation may not be the appropriate or useful one. However, policy is built on values and Medicare policy values medical convalesence, not support care for the chronically ill.

Part of that value clearly was based on cost. The framers of Medicare viewed medical care and health care as the same thing; therefore home health care would be home medical care. Services that are not medically directed then become nonhealth care and should not legitimately be covered under a federal health insurance program.

The other overriding concern was that by not limiting services to short-term medical ones there could simply be an unmanageable demand for subsidized room and board by the elderly. The expectation was that limiting services to medical care would hold down costs but the allowable services are the costliest and, to confound this thinking further, those expensive services are not even the ones most needed by the elderly. Policy intent and policy outcome are not always compatible.

Intermediaries and Transportation

Intermediaries' administrative costs for home health services are high. They review every bill submitted, rather than auditing just samples of billings. There are no standardized ways of reviewing and approving claims. Because home health service volume is low in relation to other Medicare services, efforts to develop more efficient methods lagged. However, regionalization of intermediaries and standardization of claim review were established belatedly.

Most home health agencies serve a given geographical community. Transportation for caregivers is an administrative problem and such expenses are reimbursable. Accessibility and safety also are administrative concerns. Most home health services are delivered in middle-class or lower-class neighborhoods that often lack public transportation or that are unsafe for lone caregivers. Escort service is difficult to provide, especially on the basis of unpredictable use. Weather presents further hazards. How to deploy caregivers for maximum travel efficiency while maintaining continuity and excellence of care is a continuing administrative headache. Home care is the only setting afflicted by these particular problems and no good solutions have been developed.

Dealing with Fraud and Abuses

Fraud and abuse also are problems in the delivery of home health services. Although less of a problem than in the Medicaid program for outpatient care, Medicare services through home health agencies have been reimbursed inappropriately (see 1977 Fraud and Abuse Amendments, P.L. 95-142 and DHEW,

April 1979). Whereas the overuse or inappropriate use of Medicaid outpatient services would benefit the providers (especially individual physicians), similar overuse or inappropriate use of Medicare home health care is also determined by providers (nurses), but they gain no direct benefits. Instead it is most often the patients who tend to receive benefits, such as needed care, even if it is not allowed.

Since home health services are based on costs and physician reimbursement is based on charges (which are not cost related) there is far greater potential for economic gain in payments to physicians rather than to agencies. Although the proprietaries represent only 15 percent of all home health agencies, they account for 21 percent of all Medicare money spent on home services and relatively more often are found to be claiming reimbursement fraudulently than are voluntary or public agencies (DHEW, November 1979). The categories of fraud and abuse include:

- billing for services not provided
- misrepresenting services
- altering bills and receipts
- duplicating billings
- falsifying records or documents
- certifying fraud
- padding payrolls
- allocating costs improperly
- violating interim payment rates

QUALITY: DEFINING AND ASSURING IT

Quality issues are particularly difficult to address in home health services. As in almost all health care settings, there is no consensus on what constitutes quality in home services:

- Is quality providing the services most superior technologically and personnel most highly trained?
- Is quality providing what most satisfies the patients?
- Is quality care aimed at increased longevity?

Home care quality depends first on the goal the service is supposed to achieve. Health care professionals in all settings want to provide the very best care available and regard cost as secondary. Quality therefore becomes equated with the very best care available and whether that service is needed or appropriate may not always be a deciding factor.

The second issue—that quality should be a factor—is particularly necessary in federally funded health care because there is accountability to the taxpayers as well as to the beneficiaries of the services.

The third major problem in quality is peculiar to home care. It involves the split accountability for the services and the isolated setting for care delivery. Physicians are held responsible for referring patients to home care, for certifying the need for allowable services, and for ordering that care. The care also must follow an episode of illness or injury. But the care is given in the home, where physicians' services are nearly unknown today and concerns needs about which doctors tend to have little knowledge.

To make the accountability even more elusive, it is not the physicians but the nurses (or other professional therapists) who give the care. It is the hallmark of professionals that they be accountable for their actions, knowing not only how to perform something but also why, when, and for what purpose. Although nurses provide physician-ordered care in hospitals, the doctors are present at least part of the time, not only to assess their patients' true needs but also to work out treatment plans with the nurses. If a nurse decides to ignore or change a physician's plan, that becomes known and must be justified or rectified.

In home care the situation is very different. Not only are the physicians planning services for unknown settings and needs but also have little or no knowledge of what care actually is given. Neither do any other professionals because home visits generally are solo visits and only the therapist and the patient know what occurs. Lack of oversight not only may lead to poor measurement of quality but also may hamper its development because the practitioner has no peer review or collaborative learning experiences.

THE ROLE OF THE MARKET

The market for home health services is complex. In general, it is not a free market since the buyers know very little about the product and therefore cannot make knowledgeable choices and the providers (physicians, primarily) control both supply and demand. These points are true in home health services as well. In addition, the market, as with nursing homes, is dominated by a single buyer—the government. This dominant buyer wields enormous power over the supply of services by dictating reimbursement, eligibility, and even service development funds. And, again, the buyer is not the user of services.

All of these factors make it very difficult to predict utilization or to know whether the product delivered is meeting the needs of the beneficiaries. Furthermore, overdemand for home services results in different outcomes than in other areas of health care delivery. Institutional care is limited by bed availability. If a bed is available, the other services also are available—dietary, linen, and housekeeping as well as laboratory, x-ray, and all of the technology and personnel required for a full range of care. If a bed is not available, none of those services can be provided. It's all or none so it is quite easy to measure who in a community is receiving care and who is not.

Home health services work differently. The resources are just as finite and discrete but patients do not receive them on an all-or-none basis. With increased demand for services, the additional patients are accepted for care but each then will receive fewer services per visit or fewer visits.

For example, home health aide service usually is provided below the level of demand so the agency will not have to pay salaries for which there is no utilization and no reimbursement. If demand for aide services increases, patients may receive fewer hours of service a week; if demand for nursing service grows, patients will have fewer nurse visits or less comprehensive nursing care. In this way, even if care is so meager as to be inadequate, a community may appear to be well provided with home health services.

This flaw is compounded by the finding noted earlier that home care is provided in isolation from observation and in the absence of clear criteria for quality. It would be most unlikely for institutionalized patients to receive such care changes as these in relation to resource availability. Whole floors of hospitals have been closed to admissions if staff there is inadequate to give all needed care.

The market for home health services suffers also from the lack of a proper reimbursement model. Charges for services depend on the caregiver employed, with nurses reimbursed at the highest level, then the other professional services, and finally home health aides at the bottom of the scale. Each professional service is reimbursed per visit, whether it lasts ten minutes or two hours, although there are agency guidelines that set expectations for the length of a visit (less than an hour and no longer than an hour and a half, for instance, for a nursing visit). Allowable costs calculated in a professional visit include transportation time to and from each patient's home and time for documentation.

The true cost of any number of different nursing services is not known since one fee covers one or all. Excluded from direct service costs, and included only as an allowable ''administrative'' expense, are the services of a nutritionist as well as nurse assessment visits to patients to determine their need and eligibility for care. Both of these types of administrative visits constitute professional health care services. Nonprofessional visits (e.g., home health aides) are charged and reimbursed by the hour.

All home health services today are a reflection of Medicare policy. Nearly three-quarters of home health agency revenues are from Medicare's coffers. There are nearly 3,000 certified home health agencies—twice as many as in 1963, pre-Medicare. Of the home health agencies, 85 percent are public or voluntary; 15 percent are proprietaries (DHEW, Nov. 1979).

These problems of cost, use, quality, and market complexity create concern for administration of home health services: how to predict need for services, how to supply and charge for them, and how to monitor quality, utilization, and cost. These are problems for policymakers as well because proper and efficient use of public funds demands knowledge of how the health care system works—knowledge that is incomplete and vague in the area of home services.

REFERENCES

Bellin, L. Personal communication, October 18, 1972.

Berkman, L., & Syme, S. Social networks, host resistance and mortality: A 9-year study of Alameda County residents. *American Journal of Epidemiology,* November 1979, *109,* 186-204.

Community Health Services and Facilities Act, 1961.

Fox, P., & Clauser, S. Trends in nursing home expenditures: Implications for aging policy. *Health Care Financing Review,* Fall 1980.

Hammond, J. Home health care cost effectiveness: An overview of the literature. *Public Health Reports,* July-August 1979, 305-311.

Editorial. *Health Care Financing Review,* Fall 1980.

Home Care in New York State. Albany, N.Y.: Home Care Association of New York State, May 1979.

Home health services under Titles XVIII, XIX, & XX. Department of Health, Education, and Welfare, Report to Congress, April 1979.

Home health and other in-home services. Department of Health, Education, and Welfare, Report to Congress. November 1979.

Leahy, K.M., Cobb, M.M., & Jones, M.C. *Community health nursing.* New York: McGraw-Hill Book Company, 1972.

Medicare Home Health Agency Manual, HCFA. Contains transmittal letters from HCFA to HHAs to define compliance as new regulations are written.

Medical Assistance for the Aged Act (Kerr-Mills), 1960.

Milio, N. *The care of health in communities.* New York: Macmillan Publishing Co., Inc., 1975.

New York Times editorial, "Medicare," July 1, 1966.

P.L. 93-641, Health Planning and Resources Development Act, 1974.

P.L. 95-142, Fraud and Abuse Amendments to 55A, 1977.

Sager, A. *Learning the home care needs of the elderly.* Waltham, Mass.: Brandeis University, Levinson Policy Institute, 1979.

Taubenhaus, L.J. Development of community health services: The physician's role. *Illinois Medical Journal,* 1965, 163-167.

U.S., Congress, House, Committee on Ways and Means, Hearings on H.R. 4222, 87th Cong., 1st sess., 1961.

Vladeck, B. *Unloving care.* New York: Basic Books, Inc., 1980.

Weissert, W. Effects and costs of day care and homemaker services for the chronically ill. National Center for Health Services Research, February 1980.

Chapter 5

Policy Guidelines and Professional Decision Making

Medicare has shaped home care policy and services to an extraordinary degree. Patient eligibility and kinds of services allowed are highly regulated. (P.L. 89-97 Sec. 1861(m) is the Medicare section on home care eligibility.) Physicians must certify these requirements for every patient whose care is reimbursed by Medicare.

Once admission to service has been achieved, however, little is required (or known) about actual delivery of care in the home. This is primarily because the setting, the patient's home, isolates the caregiver from the peer consultation or supervision that characterizes other clinical care. This isolation results in lack of public knowledge about the content of care and the rationale for services provided. The documentation in patient records and on billing forms is meant to reflect the care actually given but there still is tremendous latitude for other services (perhaps unreimbursable ones).

This is particularly true when two different professionals, such as physician and nurse, are involved. The physician writing the orders has a perspective on health care that is based on acute illness and curative services—the medical specialty. However, the physician knows relatively little about the development of adaptation, support, and assistance required in the home to carry out a medical plan. When the nurse implements the physician's plan, a number of changes or additions may occur, some adaptive, others caused by a difference in perspective.

Nurses value medical care, and assist in carrying it out in all settings but they also value their own autonomous services aimed at improving or maintaining health and preventing disease or disability. Their care may be expected to encompass these other areas, especially in the home, where there is a great deal of freedom to determine what service to provide during any given visit to a patient.

These two potentially conflicting factors, well-developed policy and a high degree of professional autonomy, make Medicare home health services a particularly rich area for research.

HOME CARE RESEARCH STUDY

The following presentation is drawn from the author's research study of the impact of professional decision making on the implementation of Medicare home care policy (Mundinger, 1981). The study involved observation of 50 home visits to Medicare beneficiaries who had no other insurance coverage. A voluntary home health agency in the northeast was utilized. The agency is divided into 12 care groups of three or four nurses each. Each group is responsible for patient care in a distinct geographical community within the agency's service area. The patients visited represented each geographical and ethnic community in the service area.

The nurses observed represented each care group and were observed for one full day apiece. They were chosen on the basis of who had the most Medicare-only visits planned on the day of observation in that particular care group. All care was recorded. At the end of each observation day the care given was compared with the three major Medicare eligibility criteria:

1. The patient must be homebound.
2. The patient must require skilled care.
3. The patient must have a physician's written plan for that skilled care.

This information then was analyzed to determine whether patients were eligible for the care they received and, if not, why the nurses continued to provide it.

ELIGIBILITY FOR HOME CARE

Homebound, as defined in the Medicare regulations, "is the normal inability to leave home; leaving home would require a considerable and taxing effort." Patients can remain eligible if they leave home infrequently so long as those trips are to receive medical care. The regulations add: "Homebound is usually defined as being caused by illness or injury."

Skilled care has changed in meaning since passage of the Medicare act in 1965 but all Medicare definitions are far more limited than the way the term is understood in general usage. Skilled care, as defined by Medicare, initially meant hands-on nursing for the resolution of the medical condition that qualified the patient for services in the home. That limited care to only tasks related to the qualifying condition. If a patient needed other hands-on care for another prior and continuing condition, that did not qualify.

The definition of reimbursable skilled care has since been expanded to include teaching as well as hands-on service, provided the teaching is necessary for the medical resolution of the primary condition. Hands-on care for other medical conditions also is covered provided that it, too, is necessary for the recovery process of the primary condition. An example would be exercises for long-standing arthritis debility for a patient convalescing from a stroke.

Even the more liberal Medicare definition does not cover important elements of care considered skilled by the practitioners involved. For example, illness prevention, health promotion, and maintenance care are disallowed even though of a highly professionally skilled nature.

Only convalescent care following an acute episode of illness is covered by Medicare; the cost of chronic care would have been prohibitive. Since only part of the full scope of needed service could be financed, acute care was chosen because this was causing the biggest financial problems, both for the elderly and for the hospitals when the elderly could not pay their bills. The strongest and most effective opposition to Medicare passage, the AMA, also was more supportive of a program geared toward physician-directed treatment of acute illness. Skilled care therefore means physician-directed care for limited conditions.

The plan for care, the third requirement for Medicare eligibility, is to be developed by the referring physician and is to be used by the nurse as the definitive guide for service given. The plan must involve services allowable under Medicare (skilled care). Homebound status and need for skilled care also must be certified by the referring physician.

Home care eligibility under Medicare is meant to limit service to only conditions that otherwise would require hospitalization. Health needs of the elderly were not the priority in the planning for Medicare home health services; the focus instead was on solving the financial problems incurred.

Of the three criteria, homebound status and skilled care relate to patients' characteristics; only the care they need and their ability to leave home are measured and discussed. Because each patient presents different characteristics, care obviously is implemented in a highly individualized manner. In direct contrast, the third criterion—physician-directed care—has no requirement that it be linked to the patient's condition. It is purely a process-oriented criterion: the physician must establish, sign, and review the plan of care to be given by nurses. Nowhere is there any requirement that the physician's care, or the plan, be appropriate, of high quality, comprehensive, or even adequate.

In the analysis for this study, however, the adequacy of the physician's plan was measured, even though Medicare does not require it, so that it could be determined whether the plan's adequacy was a factor in nurse decision making about care provided.

Case studies were developed for all 50 patients and those that illustrated particular themes are discussed here and in Chapter 6. The cases illustrate the wide variety of home environments and support systems for the elderly and provide the background the nurses used in making decisions about the care they would deliver (Mundinger, 1981).

SKILLED CARE: EFFECTIVE SERVICE LIMITATION?

Everyone concerned with reimbursement decisions agrees that the skilled care criterion is the most important one for Medicare eligibility purposes. Nurses and administrators in the study agency universally named skilled care as the most important qualifier in their documentation for reimbursement. The individuals who review claims and make reimbursement decisions in the intermediary office also state that this criterion plays the major role in determining coverage eligibility.

Because it is so important, and is increasingly broadly interpreted, it is interesting that nearly a third of the patients visited (16 out of 50) did not meet the skilled care conditions. All 50, however, initially had met this criterion on admission to home health care and in each case those services still were being delivered during the observed visits. For the 16 exceptions, those services no longer were needed and thus no longer qualified as skilled. For purposes of reimbursement and continued access to service, however, the nurses continued to claim those services as skilled.

The following patients are good examples of the exceptions.

Case 1: Mrs. Pietro Castaldo

Mrs. Pietro Castaldo, who is 85 years old, lives with her husband in a tiny, immaculate house. She had been hospitalized recently with a concussion following a fall on an icy street. During her hospitalization her blood pressure fluctuated between normal and above-normal range. After discharge, she was followed at home for cardiovascular monitoring. Her blood pressure was stable and her medication regime set. However, she needed other care.

Following the enforced bed rest for her concussion, she had developed chronic constipation and her previously arthritic knees were causing constant pain and immobility. The day of her visit she was suffering from frequent diarrhea and rectal discomfort. The nurse spent nearly an hour relieving the patient's impaction, then spent time with her and her husband going over a diet that could prevent further episodes of severe constipation. Range of motion and heat to her knees were provided and the nurse also reviewed Mrs. Castaldo's ambulation with a walker.

The woman's blood pressure was up slightly at the beginning of the visit, which helped to justify the nurse's continuing visits that were serving a necessary, if maintenance, function. At the end of the visit, with the patient comfortable and relieved of her anxiety, the blood pressure was again in her normal range.

A maintenance regime was being established for Mrs. Castaldo to aid her in regaining stability at home. Her husband, who will continue to care for her, needs the nurse's teaching and support as well. Although unrelated to her medical crisis, the care being given may prevent rehospitalization.

The nursing care and support provided to this family allowed for the patient to be cared for at home. Each of the 15 other exceptions to reimbursable care was receiving similar needed services. Two patients provide further examples.

Case 2: Mrs. Lettie Woods

Lettie Woods is a 67-year-old black who lives alone in an apartment in "the projects"—a low-income, noisy building. She is one of only two patients of the 50 who had not been hospitalized before referral for care. Blind and hypertensive from long-standing diabetes, Mrs. Woods was referred by her physician who had become frustrated with lack of success in managing her care. His orders read, in their entirety:

management diabetes
control hypertension
visit q week—monitor vital signs, med administration
lo sodium—lo sugar

Her medications were listed, with dosages: two hypertensive medications, iron, a diuretic, insulin, and a stool softener. Since she cannot see, Mrs. Woods identified her medication bottles by different sets of rubber bands. The nurse found that a grandchild who visited regularly played with the pill bottles, pulled at the rubber bands, and mixed them up. Part of Mrs. Woods's medication problem was linked to this.

Because the physician wanted Mrs. Woods maintained on home care and "not in my office," he changed medications for her every so often so there would be justification for continued Medicare coverage (Medicare will not pay for maintenance service, only for care that promotes change). Therefore Mrs. Woods had numerous bottles of hypertensive medications, in varying dosages, and she forgot which were the current ones. These two factors led to medication noncompliance.

The nurse was able to arrange a more reliable and safe medication procedure on this observed visit and during this period of observation for "unstable blood pressure" the nurse continued to visit to assure a safe environment, proper nutrition and to help Mrs. Woods document her medication and other medical expenses so that she could qualify for Medicaid. Medicaid eligibility would then allow for maintenance services, such as a homemaker, which was her primary need.

Case 3: Tess Muldoon

Tess Muldoon, 70 years old and recently widowed, while recovering from a hip replacement contracted pneumonia. She was rehospitalized and when ready to come home again her physician's orders included a request for the same nurse, by name, who had cared for Mrs. Muldoon previously. Although the qualifying episode for this period of home care was pneumonia, the physician's complete orders were:

continue to ambulate with crutches
eval. home health aide bid
cough med—very anxious

Although ambulation and home health aide services were accomplished easily, the nurse's real goal was to provide psychological support, continuity, and assure proper nutrition and sleep during her time of convalescence. Mrs. Muldoon was moving to a new apartment in a new neighborhood after 20 years in the same house. The stress of recent widowhood and illness and moving was being ameliorated by her nurse. It was the resolving pneumonia, however, that justified the visits.

The nurse was well aware of what she was doing in these visits, and how she was using the pneumonia as a legal basis for her care. She was even continuing to see the patient at her new address although it was out of her geographical area.

When all 16 exceptions to skilled care policy were studied it became apparent that nonreimbursable care fell into three distinct categories: counseling, teaching, and health maintenance:

1. *Counseling* is defined as planned nursing interaction in which patients develop or strengthen new attitudes or new beliefs that enable them to carry out prescribed therapy or life style changes. For example, patients may accept a new self-care regime based on the belief that it will not adversely affect their self-image.

2. *Teaching* is defined as planned nursing intervention in which patients acquire a new motor skill or new knowledge (e.g., teaching a new diet regime or teaching a patient to do exercises). Teaching new diabetics their diet and how to give their own insulin is reimbursable care; diet teaching to relieve constipation for a diabetic, however, is not reimbursable. Only teaching for the resolution of the specific medical problem is considered skilled.

3. *Health Maintenance* is defined as activities other than teaching or counseling that prevent illness or maintain the health of the patient. Such activities include providing comfort and safety, therapeutic changes such as modifying diet, referrals for new services and coordination of existing ones, and nursing assessment and care to assure that a patient can function as independently as possible in routine self-care. The services are aimed at maintaining each patient at the highest level of independent and healthful functioning.

It is apparent from these definitions that care that is reimbursed as skilled depends on the conditions under which it occurred. These are situational definitions. Therefore, a component of care must be seen in the context of the patient's medical condition before it can be considered reimbursable or nonreimbursable. Although none of the 16 patients who were exceptions to the criteria were receiving care defined as skilled under Medicare law, each was in fact obtaining service that was needed (Table 5-1). Furthermore, the "illegal" care was reimbursed because skillful documentation by the nurse in each instance linked the service given to a convalescent medical need.

The nonreimbursable services delivered to all patients were remarkably similar. This indicates that all of these particular older patients' requirements for health services in the home were similar and were not dependent on their needs for skilled care. For instance, Mrs. Muldoon was receiving nutritional and exercise care to prevent another episode of pneumonia. This suggests that limiting care to recuperative services may be unworkable.

There were important differences between the eligible and ineligible populations. The reimbursable care population received dressings twice as often as cardiopulmonary monitoring and the 16 patients who were exceptions to the criteria received just the opposite. It follows that the need for cardiopulmonary monitoring may be easier to claim than the need for dressings. This may be because cardiopulmonary changes often are labile and impermanent and therefore can be claimed more easily to be present whereas conditions requiring dressings are more verifiable. Another possible explanation of why cardiopulmonary monitoring is unreimbursable care is that it is less likely to be linked to a changeable medical condition than dressings; therefore, even if the monitoring is needed, it may not meet skilled care criteria. Here is such a patient.

Table 5-1 Nonreimbursable Nursing Services Delivered to Reimbursable and Nonreimbursable Care Patients

Types of Care*	Reimbursable Care Patients (N = 34)		Nonreimbursable Care Patients (N = 16)	
Health Maintenance	33	(97%)	16	(100%)
Teaching	29	(85%)	13	(81%)
Counseling	22	(65%)	12	(75%)

*Some patients received multiple services of counseling, teaching, and health maintenance.

Case 4: Lorraine Baltimore

Lorraine Baltimore is an 83-year-old black living alone in a dark, cluttered apartment on the top floor of a frame house in the downtown area. She is tall, thin, and gracious. She once was a master seamstress and her beautiful old Singer machine shares a spot in the dining room with a framed "Trade Dressmaker" certificate. Two months earlier she had broken her hip. It was pinned and she was sent home to ambulate with crutches and without weight bearing.

Both Mrs. Baltimore and the nurse have been unable to reach the orthopedist for an appointment or even for verbal instructions regarding weight bearing. The nurse visits her to monitor her ambulation safety and to provide range of motion to her hip. Mrs. Baltimore has long-standing diabetes and hypertension so the nurse justifies continued Medicare coverage on the basis of the patient's unstable blood pressure and recurring chest pains.

A second clear difference between the two groups of patients was the underlying reason for care (Table 5-2). For the 16 patients who were exceptions to eligibility, half had chronic disease as the underlying cause for care and half had trauma and other acute illness. Of the patients receiving reimbursable care, 82 percent had chronic illness as the underlying reason for service.

Although the intent of the statute is specifically to cover convalescent costs of short-term acute illness, this finding indicates that the majority of reimbursable care arises from chronic disease. Conversely, unreimbursable care needs more often were the result of acute illness or trauma.

Table 5-2 Underlying Reason for Home Health Services

	Reimbursable Care Patients (N = 34)	Nonreimbursable Care Patients (N = 16)
Chronic Disease	28 (82%)	8 (50%)
Trauma and Acute Illness	6 (18%)	8 (50%)

Elderly persons convalescing from acute illness may be more in need of custodial or maintenance service than care aimed specifically at resolution of the medical problem. What may happen is that patients gain access to Medicare home health services because of an acute illness episode but the care they receive at home is primarily health maintenance.

These findings emphasize the contradiction in Medicare policy and actual home care practice. It is the chronically ill who are receiving the majority of services while those who need care because of an acute episode are not getting reimbursable treatment much of the time.

Another important difference between the reimbursable care patients and those who were exceptions to policy was the living arrangement for each group (Table 5-3). Half of the ineligible patients lived alone as compared to slightly more than 25 percent of the eligible ones; patients living alone thus were nearly twice as likely to receive ineligible care. This finding suggests that living alone may be a factor that explains why nurses keep patients on service after their care eligibility lapses.

The skilled care criterion is the one nurses consider most important for reimbursement eligibility, yet they state that careful documentation provides a means of continuing needed care even when the service no longer is skilled. Administrators and supervisors in the agency were aware of the nurses' strategies regarding skilled care policy. A Medicare administrator said that even with broad ''professional judgment'' in interpreting skilled care, the three criteria still were doing

Table 5-3 Comparison of Living Arrangements

	Reimbursable Care Patients (N = 34)	Nonreimbursable Care Patients (N = 16)
Live with Family	25 (74%)	8 (50%)
Live Alone	9 (26%)	8 (50%)

their job in focusing care on patients who had acute medical needs. The administrator acknowledged that the skilled guidelines get stretched but however the policy might be manipulated, it still remained as a guide that limited care to short-term medical conditions more often than without such a policy.

Following are some of the nurses' comments about justifying care that no longer was skilled:

"It's semantics. If you can make it look good on paper . . ."

*   *   *   *   *

"Oh boy, that's a toughie. Sometimes the patients are eligible for Medicaid or fee adjustment but don't want to face that and won't apply. Sometimes I'll close one case and then go back once in a while as a free visit to see how they are managing. And sometimes it's just finding the appropriate wording."

*   *   *   *   *

"I try to fabricate . . . well, not really. I go in and do diet teaching, or get their safety straightened out. That's OK for a couple of visits and while I'm there I look for reasons."

*   *   *   *   *

"Oh, I find something . . . if I think they need a nurse, I make sure I find something that will satisfy Medicare."

*   *   *   *   *

"The hardest ones are those who have worked hard all their lives . . . put a little bit away . . . own their own homes . . . and so they only have Medicare and that won't pay for maintenance care. Then I have to say, 'I know you have problems but I can't help.' "

*   *   *   *   *

"I'm willing to lie for some people if they need the care."

*   *   *   *   *

"I've been able to B.S. in the chart . . . come up with something. Even in a patient without much learning potential, I'll still put down teaching

. . . maybe doing something else. I'll hang on to any skill I can find, even a small change in a med . . . or with activity, I really lay it on when a cardiac takes an extra step.''

* * * * *

''Sometimes just my intuition tells me I should be there and then I just lay it on with something I know is covered—a slight change in the sclera, an arrhythmia, anything objective.''

* * * * *

''My value system puts the person first, and his needs. The legality of something doesn't get in my way. If I felt my continued presence was needed, I'd find a way to be there—a reimbursable way.''

One of the agency administrators says: ''You can justify skilled care on paper. You can nudge it a lot and use it and do what is needed.''

A Medicare intermediary administrator approves of the skilled care criterion and accepts the broad interpretation. She said: ''Skilled care and medical direction have helped home care become more focused and appropriate. [We acknowledge that] professional judgment makes for many opinions.''

The nurses were at ease with the way they handled the criteria but also acknowledged that the policies had been helpful. One nurse who has been in public health practice for a long time explained: ''We're not just friendly visitors anymore. We used to do so many baths. Now we're working at the level where we should. Even though we don't really stay within the guidelines, we're a lot better about planning our work and giving nursing care than we used to be.''

IMPLEMENTATION IN THEORY AND PRACTICE

As discussed earlier, reimbursement for Medicare home care is based almost solely on the physician's certification of the status of the patient on admission to service. Homebound status, skilled care needs, and orders for that care all are determined by the physician. Homebound status, in fact, is inferred based on the severity of the medical diagnosis; the actual functional status need not be verified.

Once the physician certifies that admission status, patients remain eligible for service as long as the doctor's orders are updated every 30 days (this usually is based solely on the nurse's report to the physician). Rarely is eligibility questioned in the first few weeks of care.

Auditing of Billings

The weekly billings from the agencies are audited routinely by the intermediary that approves payment. If the billing does not list skilled care as what was given, the agency would be requested to give further details of the service provided to assure that it was skilled. After the first few weeks of service, audits are made more frequently—the longer the patient is on service, the more frequent and specific the audits.

Audits consist of a request from the intermediary to the agency for copies of documentation of visits made and copies of physician orders. Documentation must show how homebound the patient is in terms of the severity of the medical condition and must attest that the care provided is skilled. Usually an agency supervisor collects the needed data from the chart and from the nurse providing care.

Nurses develop individualized and comprehensive checklists that include all needed skilled care services for each patient. For example, in the care of a leg ulcer, it may list observations (size, color, and healing of the ulcer), care to be given (cleansing, débridement, topical medications, dressings), and peripheral data (swelling, coloration, pulses of the surrounding tissue). This list allows the nurse to document detailed verifying data on every visit without having to write a time-consuming narrative.

However, some care may not appear justified when only a checklist is used; in such instances, nurses do write a narrative justifying their continued care. For example, a checklist may indicate that a patient convalescing from a cardiovascular illness appears to be independent and recuperated. Blood pressure levels, color, and self-care abilities all may seem stabilized and progressively improved. However, the nurse may have noticed frequent cardiac rhythm abnormalities; or the patient may report rare, intermittent chest pain; or a recent change in medication may require renewed monitoring. These valid reasons for continued care must be in the record or payment may not be forthcoming.

Documentation of Services Provided

Nurses learn how to document care to assure reimbursment. Fabrication is rare but adjustment of the data probably is frequent. For instance, nurses may not manufacture cardiac irregularities or ulcers but they can magnify the need for eligible care in order to give needed (although ineligible) service. They may write of the one skipped beat, the barely pink healed leg ulcer, or the slightly blurred vision with great care and urgency if the patient seems to still need care.

It is interesting that this kind of documentation is entirely legal. As long as care deemed skilled actually is given, there is no required certification by the nurse that the service, or monitoring, is truly needed. As for homebound status, the nurse is not required to report the patient's actual functional status, either, but must document only the care given as ordered by the physician.

Not only is it interesting that current policy allows this professional decision making by nurses, it also is apparent that this probably does not lead to fraud and abuse. A major reason is that nurses do not receive direct payment for services but work on a salary basis for the agency. Most fraud and abuse occurs when the action directly benefits the person making the decisions. Furthermore, the frequency of home visits under Medicare is not regulated, so if nurses strictly enforced patient eligibility they still could fill their time with more visits to those patients who were fully eligible.

The Medicare Waiver

The other major check on fraud and abuse is the leverage of the Medicare waiver to home health agencies. Ineligible care, up to 2.5 percent of revenues, will be reimbursed by Medicare. If ineligible care exceeds 2.5 percent of revenues in any one year, the agency must pay for all the ineligible care that year and the waiver is denied for succeeding years.

In the case of Medicare home health care, it would appear that whatever success is achieved in substituting such services for institutionalization has occurred only through the use of so-called "skilled" treatment. In actuality, a combination of professional services brings about these outcomes and since the nonreimbursable services are indirect (or "hidden"), their contribution to the results cannot be known.

This compromises the evaluation of policy effectiveness since the services can differ substantially from what policy directs. All but one of the 50 patients received nonreimbursable services and only slightly more than two-thirds had reimbursable treatment, therefore it may be that the outcome and cost of home care depend as much, or more, on the unreimbursed segment. This would seem to be a major problem in policy evaluation and development in Medicare home health services.

HOMEBOUND: WHO REALLY KNOWS?

The second home care eligibility criterion studied was homebound status. This was determined at the time of each visit and was based on observed activity, such as seeing patients returning from a visit outside the home, or on activity they reported. Patients were not asked directly whether they considered themselves homebound but nonhomebound status was determined by information they volunteered, such as, "Please visit me in the afternoon because I go out with my friends in the morning." If nonhomebound status was suspected, the patient was asked directly, "Do you get out of the house since your illness?" Their answers were used to determine their homebound situation. Clear exceptions to homebound policy were studied further to determine what characteristics might explain why or how those patients were being continued on service.

Homebound patients fell into two groups: (1) those who were bedridden, wheelchair bound, unable to walk without assistive devices, or otherwise had medical conditions that would preclude their leaving home without considerable and taxing effort and (2) those who were physically able to leave but whose medical condition was a clear contraindication for such activity and who would be at risk for medical problems if they did go out. There is only one allowed exception to the Medicare homebound requirements: patients who need service not available on an outpatient basis, such as respiratory therapy, can receive home treatment for that care without being homebound.

Although Medicare regularly audits eligibility, homebound status is difficult to ascertain, and usually can be justified by the medical diagnosis. Medicare intermediary personnel usually base their assessment on the patient's medical diagnosis and functional condition. This often is difficult to determine since different patients with the same diagnosis can vary markedly in debility and dependence, yet their functional status usually is inferred from the medical diagnosis. No specific abilities are required to be documented.

While auditing to ensure agency compliance is their major function, intermediaries also can reverse agency decisions that they deem too limited. For instance, the intermediary for the study agency related this example: An alcoholic patient, with certifiable skilled nursing needs, living in a room without cooking facilities, walked down two flights of stairs and across the street to a diner to eat every day. The intermediary overruled the agency decision to deny services on the basis of nonhomebound status.

The Nonhomebound

Patients classified as nonhomebound were those who did not meet Medicare criteria; in each case they gave verbal reports about regular visits outside the home, and when they did leave it was not for medical treatment but for social outings. The homebound requirement is meant to limit services in the home to only those patients who otherwise would be institutionalized. If patients are not homebound, it is assumed that they can receive care in traditional outpatient areas such as clinics or physicians' offices. To assure that acutely ill patients are not discharged to home care, the qualifying criteria also state that such individuals will need "intermittent" skilled care. The intent of the intermittent care provision is to limit such service to convalescents or the less acutely ill.

Even with this major qualifier, nearly 40 percent of the patients studied were not homebound. This is not an indication of negligent observations by the nurses, for they were well aware of which patients were not homebound and did not document their real status. This was a deliberate strategy for the nurses and, as one said, ''If you write it right, you can get away with anything.''

In the sample of 50 patient visits, every individual was considered homebound for purposes of Medicare reimbursement claims. In 31 cases, the patients were truly homebound; in the 19 others, they were not but were being cared for at home for other reasons and nurses claimed the homebound status so they could provide those needed services. The 19 who were not homebound participated in activities including attending daily mass, having season tickets to the theater, walking daily to the senior citizens center, visiting relatives, shopping, and going out for dinner or to the beauty parlor. None of them viewed themselves as homebound.

Other Operative Factors

The homebound status thus did not appear to be a valid reason for giving care in the home since nearly 40 percent of the patients were exceptions. Therefore, other factors had to be identified to provide a better explanation of why nurses chose to deliver services in the home rather than discharge patients who no longer met eligibility criteria. All services to patients were identified and the reasons for giving care in each case were examined. It became clear that two categories were involved (Table 5-4):

1. In more than half of the visits, home resources were being adapted and utilized in the delivery of services to patients.
2. In the observed nursing visits, two-thirds of the patients received multiple services that are not available in any other single care setting.

Table 5-4 Factors Associated with Giving Care in the Home

	Homebound Patients (N = 31)	Nonhomebound Patients (N = 19)
Adaptation of Home Resources Necessary for Care Given	17 (55%)	9 (47%)
Multiple Services Delivered Not Available in Any Other Single Setting	22 (71%)	10 (53%)
Patients Receiving Care in at Least One of These Categories	24 (77%)	14 (74%)

NOTE: Some patients in each category received both types of care.

Where adaptation of home resources is required for services, it makes sense that the care is delivered and taught most appropriately and efficiently in that setting.

As for multiple nursing services, they were ones that could not be delivered in any single outpatient visit. For example, a patient whose home care was being directed by a surgeon for diabetic ulcer care could not obtain diabetic diet management or disability counseling in that physician's office. In a hospital, the multiple services are available, but only through the visits of a variety of professionals; the dietitian for diet assistance, the social worker for counseling, and physiotherapists or occupational therapists to devise ways of carrying out exercise or self-care.

Even though physiotherapy and occupational therapy are covered under Medicare home health benefits, the nurse was providing those services or counseling or nutritional assistance for nearly two-thirds of the patients observed.

Both the truly homebound patients and the 19 exceptions to policy received care in multiple services and home adaptation. Slightly more of the homebound than the nonhomebound patients were represented in these categories, which perhaps reflects their needs as a result of being truly homebound. Even though less often represented in these categories, the nonhomebound may have been maintained on home care because of these two categories of need. Two examples follow.

Case 5: Mrs. Giuseppe Franco

Mrs. Giuseppe Franco is 70 years old, Italian speaking, and lives with her daughter and three granddaughters in a small house high on a hill in a residential area. The house is immaculate and Mrs. Franco, in matriarchal splendor, is ensconced in the parlor-TV-dining room. She has on a black dress, black sweater, and black slippers. Her gray hair is in a neat bun and covering her lap is a crocheted lap rug. She has a religious medal pinned to her bosom and her foot with the ulcer is elevated on a stool.

It is Saturday morning a week after New Year's and Mrs. Franco's daughter is in the kitchen making pastries. Four kinds already are on the counter, and she is frosting a cake.

Mrs. Franco is a diabetic and had developed an ulcer on her ankle and cellulitis of the leg requiring hospitalization. Now she is home, the ulcer is healing, and the cellulitus has resolved. Two of her major concerns are getting to mass every day and preventing constipation.

She can't wait to sample the pastries, which gives the nurse the opportunity to review the diabetic diet with the daughter. Mrs. Franco is wearing half stockings with elastic just below the knee, clearly contraindicated in a diabetic with peripheral vascular insufficiency. Again, this presents an opportunity for health teaching. The dressing is accomplished with all three granddaughters watching so they can help later.

Homebound? No, but there is no one place such a patient can go for both dressing changes and health teaching. A visit to her surgeon's office for the dressing change would require a ten-mile round-trip cab ride or walking four blocks down the steep, icy hill to wait for the bus. Going to mass is easier. The church is only two blocks away, on a level with their house, and her granddaughters accompany her before they leave for school.

Case 6: Mrs. Patrick Fisher

Mrs. Patrick Fisher is 69 years old, Irish, and lives in a small apartment on the sixth floor of a seedy brick apartment building. She has wispy white braids on top of her head and her dress is very large for her because she has lost 100 pounds in the last year.

She has a colostomy as a result of surgery for diverticulitis and traditional care is not working because the stoma has no handy ring of tissue on which to place a colostomy bag. Instead, the opening is recessed and it has taken a good deal of consultation and creative technology on the part of the nurse to get a good fit.

Mrs. Fisher frequently goes shopping and down to the third floor to visit her sister, who has an apartment there. Mrs. Fisher requires a special diet because of her diverticulitis and recently has developed severe ankle edema.

Part of the success in home care for Mrs. Fisher is attributed to the use of home resources and important observations made by the nurse. Diet teaching was initiated for both the diverticulitis and sodium restriction for the ankle edema. In the tiny cramped bathroom, the sink overhangs the toilet for a few inches and Mrs. Fisher could not carry out her colostomy care there, so a simple and efficient method was devised in the bedroom. The nurse even obtained additional supplies through Medicare to make this possible. The nurse made an appointment for Mrs. Fisher to see her medical doctor about the ankle edema.

Homebound? No, but again there was no one place Mrs. Fisher could go for assistance in diet teaching and colostomy care. If she were to return to her surgeon for this, would he be likely to look for and treat ankle edema? And what about diet teaching? Where could a patient be referred for that?

Another patient, suffering from malabsorption related to progressive systemic sclerosis, was being maintained on hyperalimentation at home. All of the home adaption required for this complex procedure had been accomplished by the nurse.

On one observation day, three of the four patients visited clearly were not homebound and the nurse discussed that problem: "Usually I just ignore their outings and make sure I don't chart them. Some services aren't available other places or, if they are, the patient just isn't mobile enough to get there or doesn't have the money."

A major part of the problem for many of the elderly who might get care elsewhere is money. Medicare does not cover transportation costs and outpatient care is subject to partial payment, whereas home care is fully covered, and the only transportation required is the nurse's—which Medicare does cover. Furthermore, these services would not have been as specific or helpful if delivered outside the home because the patients needed to understand how to use their own resources in their own homes in order to accomplish self-care effectively and safely.

The nurses were conscious of their handling of the homebound requirement and not surprised that such a large percentage of their patients was not really homebound. Sometimes the patients made it more difficult for nurses to comply with Medicare policy. In one instance a patient being seen for daily care of leg ulcers refused to acknowledge that she was supposed to be homebound, saying:

"You think I'm a gonna stay home? What am I gonna stay for? What am I gonna do here? I have a big family. I see them. I go here, I go there. They come and get me. Why I wanna stay home? I'll be here when you come, but I not gonna stay here."

A third factor associated with nonhomebound patients was their living arrangement. As with the skilled care category, patients living alone were far more likely to continue receiving home health services after their eligibility lapsed than those who lived with family (Table 5-5).

In the patients studied, some who were severely dependent lived with family but others equally dependent lived alone. The absence of family made a difference in how long home care services were supplied but there was no observable relation between dependency level of the patient and lack of family. This was a surprising finding for it might seem logical that severely dependent patients would be accepted for home care services only if the family support systems were adequate to assure their safety.

One patient living alone was bedridden and from 5 o'clock each evening to 9 o'clock the next morning was completely by herself. Her greatest fear was that she would end up in a nursing home and she refused institutionalization, saying she was determined to die before that could happen.

Table 5-5 Relationship between Living Arrangement and Homebound Status

	Homebound Patients (N = 31)		Nonhomebound Patients (N = 19)	
Live Alone	7	(23%)	10	(53%)
Live with Family	24	(77%)	9	(47%)

Case 7: Adeline Drago

Adeline Drago is small, sweet faced, and white haired. She is 83 years old and had been hospitalized for four months after her nieces found her sick in her apartment, dehydrated, without food, and unable to care for herself. Once she began to recover, plans were made with the nieces to provide for her safe care at home.

Although old and ill, Mrs. Drago still was in command of her mental faculties and she had made it clear to everyone that she would use her carefully saved money to hire the help necessary so she could stay in her own home.

What happened after that is unclear, but the homemaker who has been with her during the day since her discharge from the hospital tells the nurse that the nieces stole Mrs. Drago's bankbooks, deposited them in some way so that there no longer is any record of Mrs. Drago's money, and that the nieces now are being increasingly niggardly about the care they are willing to fund for her. First, they cancelled the night aide, then the evening one. Now only this one young homemaker stands between Mrs. Drago and death. She needs help in feeding herself, she cannot care for her catheter, and she cannot dial the phone by her bedside. She cannot turn the light switch so she sits all night in darkness, or under the light, depending on her preference at 5 o'clock.

She lies uncomplaining in her hospital-type bed, surrounded by plastic flowers and year-old Christmas cards. She has a tiny stuffed animal that she keeps in bed with her, and she wears a satisfied smile as she eats Jell-O and watches television.

The nurse discussed her dilemma: Should she go to court to get Mrs. Drago round-the-clock care as a matter of safety? If so, wouldn't the patient just end up in a nursing home? Should a nurse protect someone's life by destroying its quality? The nurse said that for now she would continue to "pop in on her during my lunch hour" (as a "free" visit) and keep an eye on her safety that way. (This case is discussed further in Chapter 6.)

THE LIVE-ALONES AS SPECIAL CASES

Nurses recognize that they make a special case for patients who live alone. The agency supervisor noted that the biggest problem she saw in the delivery of care was "the borderline patient, the elderly person without interested others, someone who needs a caretaker or at least some supervision, and they are not eligible for service. Medicare, if you want to know the truth, is a barrier. It is fine to open a case but there are no supportive services. Nurses learn to document to get services covered but Medicare just won't pay after the restorative goals have been met."

Another nurse told of a patient who lives alone:

"She's a cardiac patient and, after one of her crises, I visit her when she goes home. She won't spend any of her money for maintenance care once Medicare stops, she thinks she's entitled. Then she has one of her scenes—her doctor calls her the second Sarah Bernhardt—and gets herself all upset and back in the hospital. Then, of course, I can go back and visit her again for a while."

When asked how the decision concerning the frequency of visits is made, many nurses responded, "I see a patient more often if there is no family." Another nurse said:

"I may go in extra on a Friday so they will be ready for the weekend." Still another nurse tells this story: "I have a patient, an old woman, tall and heavy, discharged home after a hip fracture. She lives alone, can't get out of bed by herself, and I couldn't place a home health aide with her by the time she was discharged home. I go in that day and the woman is incontinent in bed because she can't get out. I try to reach some of her family and that doesn't work because there is some kind of feud going on. Then I try the landlady and we get into a fight. I could just about cry.

"All I can do is show her how to use a bedpan in bed. I worry about her all night and go in the next morning before work and find she couldn't use the bedpan so she just padded herself and went in that. She absolutely refused a nursing home but that's where she belonged.

"I certainly wasn't giving her skilled care. I just sold it to Medicare as ambulating her. We can get reimbursed for physical therapy if a therapist isn't available. So that's what I did until I got a home health aide and the therapist in. The woman made it."

Another nurse told of a woman living alone who did not make it in conventional terms:
"I get pretty involved with my patient's needs. I had one lady who lives alone and had a leaky ceiling and one weekend the ceiling fell down and she called me. I called her niece and her landlord and we got help. She had psych problems also, and sometimes she wouldn't even open the door for me. I got her psychiatrist to get her a social worker but she wouldn't let the social worker in. The only people she saw in the world were her niece, who brought groceries once a week, and me.

"One week last summer I didn't get any answer and didn't see her inside so I called the police and they found her dead, peacefully lying on a pillow in front of the air conditioner. She'd been dead about a week. I was supposedly seeing her for her heart problem but I was really seeing her because she was all alone."

Severely dependent patients are admitted to home care services whether they live alone or in a family structure. There appears to be a clear association between living arrangement and how soon a patient is discharged, however. It appears that nurses bend homebound eligibility policy more readily for those living alone and are not as likely to discharge them once they become ineligible for care. This is true even when the live-alone is not severely dependent.

ELIGIBILITY AND FAMILY PRESENCE

The findings from the analysis of both homebound and the reimbursable care policies corroborate the clear relationship between eligibility and living arrangements (Table 5-6). In each policy, half those receiving ineligible care were living alone whereas only a quarter of the eligible patients lived alone. A composite of eligibility for both policies produces findings that are even more striking: of all those living alone, only 18 percent were eligible for care. Nearly a third of the patients who lived alone (5 out of 17) were doubly ineligible, being neither homebound nor receiving reimbursable care. One is a woman who needs custodial care in order to remain independent during her convalescence.

Table 5-6 Relationship between Living Arrangement and Eligibility

	Live Alone (N = 17)	Live with Family (N = 33)
Fully Eligible	3 (18%)	19 (58%)
Ineligible for Homebound and/or Reimbursable Care	14 (82%)	14 (42%)

Case 8: Kate Donnelly

Kate Donnelly is an 80-year-old retired nurse who lives alone in a well-furnished apartment in a quiet residential area. She has a fractured humerus as the result of an automobile accident. When it occurred, she elected to be cared for at home. She is a big woman and suffers from severe osteoarthritis of both knees. She requires good arm strength to hoist herself out of her chair.

Because of the combined disabilities of the fracture and arthritis, she found she could not care for herself at home and was hospitalized. During her six-week stay two other problems became apparent: her blood pressure was unstable and she had low blood potassium. When she was discharged, it was those two medical instabilities that qualified her for skilled nursing care and, in turn, for home health aide services.

The aide is Mrs. Donnelly's real service need. The aide comes daily to bathe her, help her dress, make her lunch, assist with her exercises, help her out of her chair, and see her safely to the apartment door when her friends pick her up for a social outing.

The nurse, by providing cardiovascular monitoring, provides eligibility for aide services. The only problem is that Mrs. Donnelly no longer needs cardiovascular monitoring and is not homebound; these are claimed only so that she can have other needed services. Her nurse explains:

"I usually find my way around the regulations. I may get skilled care ordered and then go in and give other care. Oh, I find something . . . a missed beat, a dizzy spell . . . then I build on it so the documentation looks like unstable blood pressure."

Three other doubly ineligible patients needed intensive counseling.

Case 9: Vincent Grollier

Vincent Grollier is 68 years old and lives alone in a sparsely furnished apartment in an old Victorian house. He is a retired physicist and has had a lonely existence since the death of his wife. He burned his back in the shower, which is the reason for his home care.

He looks forward to the nurse's visits and follows her about as she prepares his dressing. He rarely goes out and eagerly awaits rare visitors to talk about articles in *Scientific American* or to show them old, yellowed clippings from his past. The nurse continues to see this man and apply dressings although his burn is healed.

Meanwhile, she works toward her real goal with him: to have him join a nearby senior citizen center and participate in its social functions. The patient does not seem to be in on this deception. He believes (or wants to believe) that he still requires the dressing changes. Only after he begins to participate regularly in the senior citizens program does the nurse decide to discontinue the dressings and discharge him from home care services. The day of the observed visit was the day of discharge for Mr. Grollier.

Case 10: Sally Bianci

Sally Bianci is 67 years old, living alone, and had been seen initially for dressings for an abdominal wound following a hysterectomy. Although care was fairly routine and effectively provided in a month, this woman was seen for another month because of severe psychological problems related to the surgery.

Some 20 years before, her mother had died of ovarian cancer after months of a draining abdominal wound and Miss Bianci was certain that she was being dealt the same fate. This caused severe weight loss, sleeplessness, and mental confusion.

The nurse continued to visit long after the wound was closed, reorienting the woman, calming her fears, and attempting to get her back into her previous independent life style. On the day of our visit, the patient smilingly gave us all her hoarded boxes of dressings and said, "I'll never need these again." She confided to us that she was about to go out on a date. The nurse then discharged her with goals achieved.

An important factor that seems to explain keeping ineligible patients on home care is their need for counseling. Three of the five doubly ineligible patients were seen primarily for that purpose. All of the counseling observed was aimed at helping patients cope with a new or potential disability, and providing care at home was particularly appropriate. The patients' ability to adapt and survive at home meant that the counseling had to be specific to the circumstances of each individual. When diet counseling was provided, for example, the home atmosphere was ideal because food supplies and preferences could be ascertained and utilized. Of the 19 nonhomebound patients, nine were being seen and counseled because the family and home milieu were critical to the success of the care delivered. As demonstrated earlier, both Mrs. Franco (Case 5), and Mrs. Fisher (Case 6) benefited from care in the home setting. In addition, counseling in the home can benefit the family as well as the patient.

Case 11: Alex Mendota

Alex Mendota is 62 years old and lives with his adult son in a small, neat, and attractive suburban house. Mr. Mendota's wife died of a heart attack a year ago and he believes "she killed herself taking care of me. It was right after I lost my leg." The son agrees and tells us she worked night and day to make sure everything was right for Alex.

Now Mr. Mendota has a new woman in his life, someone he met at the senior citizens center. He recently returned from the hospital where he had gone with ischemia in his remaining foot and where the surgeon had performed a sympathectomy in hopes of perfusing the foot better.

Mr. Mendota has been a diabetic for years. He also suffers from high blood pressure, gall bladder disease, and arteriosclerotic heart disease. His previous surgery for the amputation of his right leg had occurred in four separate operations, each one going a little farther up the leg until sufficient circulation allowed healing. The possibility of a second amputation now looms, for the remaining foot still is ischemic and two small gangrenous areas have formed. Mr. Mendota remembers only too vividly the year before and comments: "I've never seen a double amputee walk, right? They all have to use wheelchairs, right?"

The nurse spends considerable time going over surgical and rehabilitative care available and tells him of numerous double amputees who walk independently. She inspects the many alterations in the house Mr. Mendota has made for himself as a single amputee and praises him on his creativity and his agility. Meanwhile she spends time with the overweight son, letting him know his own health risks with two diabetic parents with heart disease and goes over exercise and nutrition tips with him.

Mr. Mendota's fiancée is a bubbly little woman with an equally optimistic personality. In fact, she assures Alex, "I just know your foot will get

better. It's all a matter of believing. You're not going to lose that foot.''
The nurse spends some time with her, too, showing her the larger areas
of gangrene and bringing Mr. Mendota's son into the counseling. Then
the three of them go through the house while she makes specific
comments about how he could continue to manage in the house and out
as a double amputee. She had even ascertained cost estimates for a car
with hand controls.

All three of these individuals received counseling from the nurse during the
observed interaction, which was the primary reason for her visit to Mr. Mendota.
    Although Medicare law requires that the homebound status must arise from the
current qualifying illness (P.L. 89-97, Sec. 1861(m)), there is no way to audit
patients' pre-illness condition. Many of the truly homebound were in that status
before their current illness.
    In the study population, more than half of the truly homebound patients (16 of
31) had been homebound previously. All still will be homebound after their current
illness episodes are resolved. In addition, seven newly homebound patients will
remain permanently homebound after the current episode.
    Thus, these 23 patients represent a group of chronically ill individuals who will
always meet at least the homebound criterion for home health service eligibility.
All they require for home health service eligibility is the need for skilled care.
    Three of the patients in this study who were homebound before their current
illnesses could have avoided expensive skilled care if preventive services had been
available under Medicare.

Case 12: James Giovanni

James Giovanni, who is 65 years old, suffered a stroke two years ago.
His devoted wife insisted on taking him home from the hospital and
caring for him herself although he was seriously incapacitated, with
movement only in his left arm. He was otherwise paralyzed, could not
speak and had a neurogenic bladder. Mrs. Giovanni set up a room on the
second floor for her husband. She got a hospital bed, learned how to care
for his catheter, and exercised his paralyzed limbs. He ate well and,
although without speech, was able to communicate his love and appreciation with expressive blue eyes, and he could squeeze her hand with
his functioning one.

After a year of this successful and loving routine Mrs. Giovanni
arranged to take a short vacation and go to Europe to visit members of
her family. Her only son, who lived in California, arranged his vacation

to coincide with hers and came to care for his father in her absence. Although well meaning and committed to this venture, the son was not as skillful or thorough in his care and his father developed four large decubiti and severe contractures during his wife's absence.

When she returned three weeks later, she was depressed and guilty to find her husband in such condition and was not able to take up his care with the same cheer and equanimity. Mr. Giovanni, however, had become eligible for home care services because of the skilled aspect of his decubiti. Under the skilled care need, the nurse now visits every two weeks and a home health aide three times a week. The aide bathes Mr. Giovanni and assists his wife in the limb exercises and decubiti care.

Mrs. Giovanni, though, says it is not the same and continues to feel guilty about her absence. Mr. Giovanni is worse off, too, and yet a home health aide or nurse during his wife's absence would have prevented the long-term, costly care now needed.

Case 13: Mrs. Leslie Trainor

Mrs. Leslie Trainor is 83 years old and has renal and retinal deterioration secondary to diabetes. Mrs. Trainor also suffers from mental deterioration from arteriosclerotic vascular disease. Her family consists of an equally vague but loving husband and an alcoholic daughter.

Mrs. Trainor is not capable of a safe and reliable self-care regime. Her recent cellulitis and renal crisis resulted from her unintentional non-compliance with her diet, medication, and activity regime. She had a hyperglycemic and hypertensive crisis, fell while trying to ambulate alone, and developed the complications that now require daily care.

Nursing visits to prevent such crises and to monitor the health of this fragile family could have been far less expensive than the costly intensive hospital and home care that became necessary.

For the permanently homebound, the reasons for their debility predictably will cause future reimbursable care needs or be used to gain access to home health services. When these elderly patients become eligible for home care, they not only gain skilled nursing but also qualify for home health aide services, which are a boon to families saddled with long-term chronic conditions. It clearly is advantageous for the permanently homebound to produce evidence of a skilled need, for then home care services can begin. These individuals also generally have chronic conditions that cause crises that justify readmission to service. Cardiovascular instability, vascular insufficiency, diabetes, and hypertension can all lead to skilled needs.

Most patients receiving home services are homebound but many are so dependent that care there poses safety risks. When Medicare criteria for home care were developed there was little concern that patients who were very ill would be cared for at home. The only attempt to limit home care to the less acutely ill was the decision to reimburse only service that was intermittent.

Unfortunately, provision of intermittent services does not necessarily mean the need is only intermittent. The regulations have evolved to set minimum limits on intermittent care: there must be at least two visits to make a patient eligible for Medicare and the time between visits cannot be greater than two months. In addition, agency policy generally limits nursing visits to no more than one a day, lasting less than an hour. Regulations limit home health aide visits to a maximum of 40 hours a week, with the average patient receiving four hours two or three times a week. These regulations provide upper and lower limits for reimbursable service and require patients to meet the minimum to qualify. However, no regulations have been developed to assure the correct level of care for patients whose need exceeds the maximum service level.

Medicare covers nursing home and hospital care, both of which usually are costlier than home service. If a patient qualifies by dependency level and need of skilled care for a nursing home or by acuteness of illness for a hospital, Medicare will pay for that higher level of care. However, patients do not follow those guidelines very well. Many fear or have a distaste for nursing homes and will do almost anything to avoid them. Some families try heroically to honor those preferences of severely dependent patients. Other families are eager to take advantage of institutional placement for a family member who has become a burden.

For the patients, and for families that want to keep a member at home, there are no reimbursable services other than intermittent skilled care. With additional services, many of the elderly could be maintained safely and satisfactorily at home and at a daily cost lower than in a nursing home. Following is a good example.

Case 14: Vincent Navarrone

Vincent Navarrone, who is 89 years old, lives with his daughter and son-in-law. He used to have his own quarters on the second floor of their house but now sleeps in the master bedroom with his daughter a few steps away on a couch and his son-in-law upstairs. Sometimes the son-in-law sleeps in a chair in the dining room to relieve his wife of care duties at night.

Mr. Navarrone is severely debilitated with cardiac decompensation and has urinary problems, blindness, esophageal abnormalities that make swallowing difficult, and cerebral ischemia. He needs nearly constant care—helping him stand to urinate, feeding him small bites of food, bathing and positioning him, helping him use oxygen at his bedside, and at night suctioning when he chokes.

Mr. Navarrone had come from Italy 60 years earlier and built the house in which he still lives. While still lucid he had extracted a promise from his daughter that he would die in his own home and she is now nearly exhausted trying to keep her pledge. Another major problem is that she recently had completed a course of chemotherapy following a mastectomy for cancer. A home health aide comes twice a week but a night attendant is also needed so this couple could have a respite from his care.

There is no money in the Navarrone family for such care; Medicare will not pay, either, but Medicare would pay for nursing home placement for this man.

Seven of the homebound patients in this study were so ill and so dependent that they qualified for institutionalization. Instead, they were at home because of the sheer determination of their families or themselves to be there. However, in one case the patient was very ill and neither she nor her family felt they could cope at home but, according to the nurse, the physician had tired of her care and had sent her home.

Case 15: Honora Maclure

Honora Maclure is a 75-year-old black who lives with her son in a small apartment. The stairs to her apartment are steep, dark, and narrow, and the catch on the door is loose. The home health aide, in slippers and baggy dress, lets us in. She is smoking a cigarette and mopping the floor in the kitchen.

We find Mrs. Maclure in the bedroom, hidden up to her eyes beneath a patchwork quilt. Her head is swathed in a bandanna. The room is dark and cold. There are two lamps but the bulbs have burned out in both. The bureau is stacked high with handbags and hats in plastic bags and there are numerous scatter rugs on the floor. Pill bottles are on a bedside table.

Mrs. Maclure had been discharged the day before after being hospitalized with osteomyelitis in her clavicle and ribs. Surgery had been done to remove the affected bones and she had a deep, draining, open wound in her chest. She also had developed decubiti on both heels, which were crusted and ready for débridement. The discharge summary noted that Mrs. Maclure's wound was "almost healed" and needed only a "dry sterile dressing" and that she had only one small heel ulcer with "no drainage." The true picture was far different, for the chest wound had profuse purulent drainage, and once the heel ulcers were débrided they were open and draining also. Mrs. Maclure also was diabetic and hypertensive. She was too weak and dizzy to sit unaided in bed, much less stand or walk. Her medication bottles were empty.

The home health aide had not yet begun to care for her and the heat in the apartment was not working this bitter cold day. The son works full time, and even the best of home health aide services rarely can be supplied for more than four hours a day. The nurse badgered the landlord into turning up the heat ("I'm not above threatening them with the Board of Health"), fired the one home health aide and hired another, had the pharmacy deliver medications, and contacted the son at work before leaving.

Of two other patients who should have been hospitalized, one was readmitted the day of the observed visit and the other died at home a week later. Of the remaining four, all of whom qualified for nursing home care, one died at home two days after the observed visit and the three others remained at home, in the care of relatives or themselves, under very precarious circumstances. One of these was Mrs. Drago (Case 7), the woman who was bedridden and alone from 5 P.M. until 9 A.M. The other follows.

Case 16: Mrs. Frederika Eaton

Mrs. Frederika Eaton is a tiny, 89-year-old lady who lives in a small apartment over a store in midtown. She is being treated for ulcers on her ankle as a result of severe, long-standing vascular insufficiency. Her other current medical conditions include arthritis, anemia, cataracts, massive hiatal hernia, congestive heart failure, chronic bronchitis, and arteriosclerotic heart disease with aortic stenosis and mitral regurgitation. What this means to the nurse delivering home care is that this woman cannot walk very well, has trouble seeing, and has both heart and lung disabilities.

When we arrive we find Mrs. Eaton in a lacy pink bathrobe sitting in a wing chair with both feet up on a kitchen chair that is at least six inches above her seat level. Her chair, the yellow couch where she apparently sleeps, and nearly every piece of furniture but the television set is covered with large blue Chux. She is very concerned that the drainage from her legs, or her own incontinent urine, will spoil the few nice things she has left.

She has a home health aide twice a week and otherwise manages for herself, including cooking and bathing. She is unable to get out of the chair without our help and we wonder how she manages on her own. She says she cooks on her gas stove, yet we read her mail to her because she cannot see the print. She cannot reach her ankles so the dressings are changed only when the nurse visits or when the home health aide comes in the afternoon two days a week.

Mrs. Eaton adamantly refuses nursing home placement although her only relative is a niece a hundred miles away. She tells us, "I don't know why God keeps me alive."

Another patient being cared for at home was a strong candidate for nursing home placement and her caregivers also were at risk because of the home care being delivered.

Case 17: Ellen Lamarski

Ellen Lamarski, an 85-year-old lady, is being cared for by her two sisters, one a retired nurse. The three women have always lived together on the second floor of an old house. The rooms are small and the wood is dark polished mahogany. Ellen had fallen and broken her hip, then developed an infection in the hip joint for which she was rehospitalized. During that stay she developed many decubiti and deteriorated mentally, no longer speaking to her visitors, becoming incontinent, and developing contractures.

Nonetheless, the sisters insisted on taking her home, regardless of their own advanced age and health problems (cardiovascular insufficiency and high blood pressure). As soon as Ellen and all her hospital paraphernalia arrived on the second floor, one of her sisters, Cecelia, developed angina and was herself hospitalized. This left Ann, the retired nurse, as the sole caregiver for bedridden Ellen. No home health aides were available immediately in the home health agency so the sisters had hired one with their own money until one could be obtained and they were very unhappy about that extra cost.

During those first few days Ann gave all the care and, in lifting and turning Ellen, developed a partially detached retina from the stress. Now Cecelia is home, mostly sitting in the kitchen drinking tea and moaning, and Ann stands by Ellen's bed, wringing her hands and getting ready for the home health aide who comes each day to turn and bathe Ellen. During our visit, Ann was taught easier ways to turn her sister that would not strain her own health.

On this visit also, the new home health aide came for the first time. She was all dressed up in a trim, double-knit pantsuit and a silky, long-sleeved print blouse. She had long, painted fingernails and dangling earrings. She looked like she was on a social visit, not a working one. She looked upset and pained by Ellen's condition and told the nurse: ''I worked in a nursing home for years but I don't work for people who can't get out of bed. I won't be able to keep working here.''

Both Cecelia and Ann are extremely at risk for their own fragile health while providing the continuous and strenuous care of their invalid sister. Only rigorous and regular services can move Ellen to a more healthful status. All three sisters clearly would benefit, in physical health, if Ellen were moved to a nursing home. But their cultural values and psychological needs forced the continuation of this risky venture at home.

HOMEBOUND STATUS LIMITATIONS

These case studies demonstrate that homebound status—that important qualifier for home health services—is not useful in limiting services to convalescents who otherwise would be hospitalized. Homebound status was meant to identify patients whose illness had caused them to be so confined and who would have been in an institution if health care were not available to them. Yet more than half of the truly homebound patients in the study had been in that position before the current episode of illness.

Although the statute requires that the homebound status be caused by the current illness, that is not so in the majority of cases studied. Only 15 of the 50 patients were homebound at the time of the observed visit *and* homebound as a result of that illness; thus, fewer than a third of those studied met both the letter and intent of the law.

Not only is the homebound status often unrelated to current illness, it also can be a permanent, continuing qualifier for home health care in much the same way that chronic disease is a permanent predictor of skilled care needs. These persons need only an acute illness with attendant skilled care requirements to be fully eligible for home health services.

While home services were meant to substitute for extended convalescent institutionalization, they can become a substitute for outpatient care instead if the patients can be claimed as homebound. The very conditions that made persons homebound put them at risk for skilled care needs: vascular insufficiencies, chronic conditions such as diabetes and hypertension, and deterioration and instability associated with old age. In other words, chronic diseases have not been omitted from Medicare home coverage but simply have been disguised as the predictable recurring crises that are caused by the chronic conditions.

Home health services are advantageous for patients not only because they carry no copayment and are unlimited in number of visits but also because they allow the elderly to receive care in their homes where they most want to be. Transportation is no problem since the care comes to the patient and many of the services provided are not available anywhere else, such as diet counseling or adapting prescribed treatment to home resources.

Because home care is so desirable and because patients must be homebound to receive it, more people may tend to be claimed as homebound (by themselves, their doctors, and their nurses) than is warranted. Homebound status is easy to create: it is inferred on the basis of the debility commonly associated with any given medical diagnosis. For instance, an elderly patient with a leg ulcer from vascular insufficiency is considered by the intermediary to be homebound, yet more than half of the patients in this study with that diagnosis were not actually homebound.

Although homebound may not work very well as a service limitation, substitute criteria to assure the appropriate use of home care services have not been developed. Without a substitute qualifier for homebound, any elderly persons with skilled care needs related to an acute illness could feel "entitled" to care in their homes even if they never were candidates for institutionalization.

FROM SUBSTITUTE TO REPLACEMENT

Without the homebound qualifier, what had been meant as a substitute for institutionalization could easily become a replacement for outpatient services. Since outpatient care requires a deductible, and copayment as well as transportation costs, and home care imposes neither expense on patients, most would opt for the latter if given the choice. Home services are very attractive to patients in terms of access and cost; homebound status, even when permanent, partially qualifies individuals for such care.

The data from this study show that more of the homebound elderly than of the nonhomebound receive nonreimbursable care. Therefore, where homebound policy is followed correctly, it may increase the utilization of Medicare home health services inappropriately. To be homebound is to be almost eligible. It is easier to find reimbursable care needs for this group because the causes of homebound status also are the qualifiers more often than for those who are nonhomebound yet do not have as high a level of functional disability.

If continuing eligibility for home health care is claimed for the permanently homebound, the chronically ill may increase their use of such services. The truly homebound may get services they do not need just on the basis of being homebound; those who are not homebound are claimed as that anyway so that other needed services can be provided (Table 5-7).

The most startling finding about homebound status was that nearly 40 percent of the patients observed did not qualify. Clearly this criterion is easy to manipulate, difficult for claims personnel to disprove, and therefore of questionable value as an effective eligibility factor.

THE PHYSICIAN'S PLAN

The third criterion studied was the one requiring a physician's plan for the services to be delivered. The interplay of the three policy criteria (homebound, skilled care, physicians' plan of care) is intended to promote doctors' direction for short-term convalescent care for patients unable to leave home. Therefore, it was important to know whether adequate physician direction for care was given. A plan was considered adequate if it covered the needed skilled care. Adequacy did not depend on the inclusion of other needed care. This limited and liberal determination of adequacy was based on Medicare eligibility; if only skilled care is allowed, then that is the only category in which to decide adequacy.

Skilled care has been defined as treatment required for resolution of the current medical problem. The majority of people over 65 have at least one chronic disease. When an elderly person is recovering from an acute illness, care of the chronic disease also must be continued and may even be the most important factor in the

---

Table 5-7 Relationship between Homebound Status and
Reimbursable Care

	Homebound Patients (N = 31)	Nonhomebound Patients (N = 19)
Reimbursable Care	20 (65%)	14 (74%)
Nonreimbursable Care	11 (35%)	5 (26%)

recovery process from the acute medical problem. The chronic care required in the resolution of the acute illness therefore is considered skilled and must be included in a physician's plan if the plan is to be considered adequate.

All but eight of the 50 patients in this study also were being treated for diabetes and/or arteriosclerotic heart disease. These conditions and their planned therapy were factors in the successful resolution of their current medical problems such as ulcers, unstable blood pressure, trauma, and surgery.

When the referral and physician's plan of care for home services are received by the agency, an initial nurse assessment visit is made within three days. The data base and revised plan of care developed by the nurse on the basis of that first visit constitutes the nurse initial assessment. When that nurse's plan is approved (signed) by the physician, it becomes the operational one for patient care and replaces the original physician order.

The plan devised by the nurse includes all of the care to be given as well as recommendations for referrals. For example, if physiotherapy is being considered as care needed, it is the nurse who makes the assessment visit to determine whether it is in fact really called for. The nurse decides on the need for a home health aide. The nurse also can make referrals for other home health services such as occupational therapy, speech therapy, and social worker services. The plan that is submitted to the physician for signature includes all reimbursable care the nurse deems necessary. It also includes illness prevention and health maintenance care required by the patient.

Of the 50 patients, 48 had a plan of care written by their physicians; the two others had no plans because their physicians had simply submitted a list of their diagnoses. After their first visit, the nurses wrote a new plan of care for each of the 50 patients and in all cases the physicians signed them, making them the official treatment plans. Some of the revisions were minor, adding only the needed but nonreimbursable tasks; others were drastic and included medical care critically needed but omitted in the physicians' plans.

Twenty-five of the 50 physicians' plans were inadequate, having omitted needed skilled care (Table 5-8). Within the group of 25 inadequate plans, a number of patterns emerge. The data reveal that care planned for primary diag-

Table 5-8 Adequacy of Physician Plan of Care by Primary and Secondary Diagnoses

	Number of Patients	Adequate Plan	Inadequate Plan
Primary Diagnosis	50	39 (78%)	11 (22%)
Secondary Diagnosis	30	15 (50%)	15 (50%)

noses was more often adequate than that outlined for secondary diagnoses. It might be expected that the most adequate care would be ordered for the primary diagnosis since that is the medical condition for which home care is ordered and predictably should be the focus of the plan. Even so, more than 20 percent of the plans for care of the primary diagnosis were inadequate.

An example of an inadequate plan for a primary diagnosis is that written for a woman with the following diagnoses.

Case 18: Florence Feiss

Congestive heart failure
Aortic stenosis
Postnecrotic cirrhosis with jaundice
S/P breast cancer (bilateral mastectomy)

Her physician's plan of care, in entirety, is:

Dr. W. to provide medical follow-up; Dr. K. gastroenterologist
Aldactone 1-2X a week
90/50—148/80
Jobst stocking
Back brace and bed board
Sk-APAP #3 1-2X a week
Dig. 0.125 mgm od
Zyloprim 300 mgm od
1500 cal 2 Gm Na diet

None of the signs and symptoms of congestive heart failure were noted to be observed or monitored, Aldactone "1-2X a week" is too vague to be an adequate order, her self-care and exercise tolerance are unknown, and her blood pressure range not addressed.

In addition, the nurse learned on her first assessment visit that Mrs. Feiss was in need of a special diet for her liver condition, that she still was jaundiced, that she had periods of disorientation, and that she was unaware of her ordered medication regime. (This case is discussed further in Chapter 6.)

Half of the plans for secondary diagnoses were inadequate. An example is Mrs. Castaldo (Case 1), who became eligible for home health services after a fall when she incurred a head injury. As that was resolved, her underlying hypertension became a problem, and home health services continued so the nurse could monitor her unstable blood pressure.

Care for secondary diagnoses also is considered necessary at times for resolution of the primary problem. Mrs. Franco (Case 5), was being seen for care of a leg ulcer but nowhere on her physician's plan of care or diagnosis list is there any evidence of her underlying diabetes and the special diet and medication that have been part of her prescribed treatment for years. During the initial visit the nurse learned of her diabetes. On the observed visit Mrs. Franco was counseled regarding restrictive elastic-top stockings and her diet was reviewed after observing her sampling the sugar-rich pastries that morning in her kitchen. The ulcer will heal faster if Mrs. Franco's blood sugar is down in a normal range and if she has no constriction to the blood vessels perfusing her legs.

Case 19: Madeline Girtner

Madeline Girtner, who is 80 years old, was discharged recently from the hospital after an acute exacerbation of chronic bronchial asthma. Her other diagnoses listed are arteriosclerotic heart disease (ASHD), paroxysmal atrial fibrillation, and severe arthritis. Her total plan of care is as follows:

Patient has chest wheezes, rhonchi, use O_2 prn
BP 108/70
Visiting nurse—monitor respiratory status
Allergic to penicillin and sulfa
Lanoxin .125 mgm OD
Theodor 300 mgm q. 12h
Lasix 40 mgm OD
K-tab 20 ml. q. 2 h.
Clinoril 200 mgm bid
Colace 100 mgm tid
Intermittent nasal O_2 3L

The nurse's initial assessment revealed that Mrs. Girtner lived alone, had two total hip replacements as the result of multiple trauma from an automobile accident 20 years before, and got around only in a wheelchair. She used a nebulizer for her lung disease, smoked cigarettes (although this worsened her lung problems), and had cataracts, glaucoma, and gout, requiring medications for the last two diseases.

The plan of care was considered adequate for her asthma (although the missing information on the nebulizer and her smoking habit might be questioned), but the important lack of information on her dependence level, other diseases, medications, and smoking made the plan inadequate for treatment of her secondary diagnosis.

If Mrs. Girtner's care had been limited to the plan, the resolution of her lung disease would have been less likely and important treatment for her other health problems would have been omitted altogether. On the day of the observed visit, Mrs. Girtner's shortness of breath was increased by the energy it took to get into her wheelchair and her decreased vision made the complex self-medication a risky venture.

Further analysis was done to see whether primary care physicians' plans differed from plans of specialist physicians (Table 5-9). This was done because referrals and plans of care of more than a third of the patients in the study (17 of 50) were developed by specialist physicians. Of those 17 specialist physicians, 14 were surgeons, two were psychiatrists, and one was a gastroenterologist. The data show that primary care physicians are far more likely to develop adequate plans of care than are specialist physicians.

Although there were only half as many specialist physicians, they developed nearly the same number of inadequate plans, or proportionately twice as many as the primary care physicians. This appears predictable for surgeons since they often meet a patient for the first time only when the person is ill with a problem requiring surgery—a fracture, a tumor, a cholecystectomy. Because of the nature of the relationship (short term, limited) a care plan that addresses the complexity of skilled care needs for that patient may not be feasible. Yet when the patient is discharged and referred to home health services, it is this specialist physician who is charged with a plan of care because the Medicare statute requires that such services ordered be for the condition that required the initial medical care or hospitalization. This case demonstrates the problem with this system.

Table 5-9 Adequacy of Plan by Primary and Specialist Care Physicians

	Adequate Plan (N = 25)		Inadequate Plan (N = 25)	
Primary Care Physicians (33)	20	(61%)	13	(39%)
Specialist Physicians (17)	5 (surgeons)	(29%)	12 (9 surgeons) (2 psychiatrists) (1 gastroenterologist)	(71%)

Case 20: Molly Goldfarb

Molly Goldfarb, who is 72 years old, fell and broke her hip while visiting her daughter. She was placed in an unfamiliar hospital and cared for by an unfamiliar surgeon. Her hip was pinned but she developed a staphylococcus infection in the incision.

When she was referred to home health services the surgeon wrote a detailed plan for changing the dressings and for physiotherapy at the house. Appropriate assistive aids (commode, wheelchair) also were ordered and the physician listed the medications Mrs. Goldfarb was allergic to (penicillin, aspirin). He discontinued her antibiotic and wrote in the chart "No meds." The care he delivered was comprehensive, high-quality surgical care, However, it was inadequate.

Mrs. Goldfarb is a diabetic and had taken Orinase for years. In addition, she has long-standing hypertension and had been taking hygroton to reduce her blood pressure. She had not taken either medication during hospitalization and when her surgeon instructed her to take "no meds" she had happily thrown out the Orinase and hygroton as no longer needed.

The nurse obtained this information on the first visit and called the primary care physician in Mrs. Goldfarb's hometown. He reordered the medications. These important medications otherwise would have been omitted for Mrs. Goldfarb's two-month recuperation at her daughter's home, and perhaps after that. Those omissions clearly could have inhibited her recovery from the infection and disabling surgery.

Nurses in this study regularly identified inadequate plans as a problem in their efforts to give high-quality care. They said physicians were unwilling to give the added information that would have allowed them to better interpret what was happening with patients, make adjustments to the plan, and make knowledgeable judgments about needed care. Some of the nurses' comments follow:

"Some patients I have problems with because they put too much strength in what the doctor says. I have this cancer patient who is also a vegetarian. The doctor wants him to build up his iron and never thinks you can get dietary iron without eating red meat. Doctors aren't as good as nurses in working around cultural differences or individual preferences. I suggested to the doctor that I could help the man get iron through a diet with eggs and other foods but do you know what the doctor said? 'The man won't eat meat because he has fat between the ears.' And the patient believes what the doctor says about only one place to get iron. So he's depressed. It gets very complicated.''

* * * * *

''I read the doctor's orders but I never decide what care I'm going to give until I see the patient. I can anticipate by their age and who they live with what they might need and their medical diagnosis. I keep the doctor advised about any changes and if I need to know more history I'll call him but usually I know what to do and I just call him to get an order changed. I have the best luck if I call and suggest what I want and they usually go along with it. If they don't agree, I just pester them until I get what I want. I had a 20-year-old man with back surgery who had a Harrington rod. Usually those patients are younger. He couldn't wash himself and was embarrassed to have his mother do it so I wanted an occupational therapist referral so he could get equipment to do it himself. This physician had never made an occupational therapist referral for a Harrington rod patient so he wasn't about to do it. He thought the guy was malingering but I talked him into it.''

* * * * *

''I like working in poor areas. I don't like the wealthier areas where everybody wants to get into the act. I have more leeway here, I can order what I want.''

* * * * *

''I usually know what I want to do. I first look at the physical problem, then the emotional . . . what do they need to help them through this? Doctors aren't helpful in determining home care needs. They're about as useful in home care as a men's room in a convent.''

* * * * *

''I think I could care for patients at home without doctors' orders—we suggest half the things our own way anyway. I've never had a referral that was accurate . . . either something is no longer done or new care isn't on the referral. I spend a lot of time checking orders and I find a lot of things that aren't on the referral, like allergies to meds, sometimes the very ones the doctor ordered! And high blood pressure . . . doctors forget that when they're treating something else.''

*   *   *   *   *

''If anything the physicians give me too much leeway . . . they rubber-stamp anything I want. I like changing meds but sometimes I have questions about what to do and they can't be bothered . . . they'll just sign off so they don't have to see the patient.''

*   *   *   *   *

''Two things make it hard for me to do what I want to do for patients. The system doesn't allow me to order even basic things —like a urine culture. And the doctors. They just don't give you the information you need. Only when patients have a real medical problem do I call them, and maybe if we had better information to begin with I could handle some of those problems too. Like this last patient we saw, if I knew what her BUN [blood urea nitrogen] is or her liver function tests maybe I would know better how to explain her behavior and how sick she really is. I called a doctor for a report of a culture last week and he wouldn't tell me. I said I was worried because the man was running a fever and you know what he said? 'Tell you what, you worry for both of us.' ''

One of the supervisors says: ''Doctors are no help in terms of policy. They think it should be paid for just because they're doctors and they ordered it. They write what they want and then complain when it can't happen. It's up to us to work around that.''

The nurses' comments showed their frustration at having physicians in charge of ordering the care they think they know better how to give. They were unhappy with the lack of interest physicians seemed to show in care given in the home and found the doctors' plans incomplete and inadequate as direction for nursing care.

In 49 of the 50 patient care records, the nursing initial assessments also identified nonreimbursable care needs not identified in the physicians' plan. In addition, care identified as needed was given in every case. It is not surprising that nurses, rather than physicians, identify nonreimbursable needs. Nonreimbursable care is preventive and maintenance as opposed to curative or rehabilitative so it is not covered often in the curative-oriented orders of a physician. The one exception in which nonreimbursable care was not identified or given was a woman who refused all interactions with the nurse except care for her foot ulcer.

Additional information nearly always was needed in order to adapt the physicians' orders to the home setting. Nurses usually obtained that information on the initial visit and used it in determining how to give care and what resources to use. For example, Mrs. Fisher (Case 6) could not do her colostomy care in her cramped bathroom and required an individualized procedure. Mrs. Woods (Case 2) was blind and needed a safe system for medication administration. Three other patients were the primary caregivers for even more debilitated family members at home so assistance was needed in planning within the family for multiple patients. In each of these cases, the nurse provided adaptation to care as well as to daily living. The adaptations included teaching other family members, devising or procuring assistive devices, and providing counseling.

One of the physician's plans that did include needed data for home adaptation was the following.

Case 21: Miss Dorothy Smith

Dorothy Smith, 60 years old, had been hospitalized recently with dizziness and chest pains attributed to a malfunctioning pacemaker. During the hospital stay, her frail sister with whom she lived died of a heart attack. Miss Smith had returned home with feelings of guilt about leaving her sister alone and with intermittent feelings of panic that the same thing might happen to her.

The nurse was to monitor her cardiovascular status and assure that the pacemaker worked well during Miss Smith's various activity levels. In the plan of care the physician included the reasons for her guilt and heightened anxiety. This added information gave the nurse clues as to how to adapt classic cardiovascular monitoring to the unique problems Miss Smith had encountered.

For 19 of the patients, however, information on home or social adaptation was missing in the physicians' care plans—details that were necessary to successfully implement the treatment program. In all cases, the additional necessary information was obtained during the initial nurse assessment visit. The needed adaptations ranged from technical tasks, specific psychological interventions, and caring for multiple patients in the home, to working with families whose resources were so meager that it was impossible to provide needed care.

Technical task adaptation was needed for Mrs. Fisher (Case 6) to be able to do her colostomy care out of her cramped and inadequate bathroom. A very complicated adaptation was accomplished by the nurse for a patient receiving daily hyperalimentation at home. In that instance the physician's order plan was very explicit about precautions and procedure but nothing had been planned for home use. That entire protocol was devised by the nurse.

In three other cases where technical tasks were combined with individual preferences and abilities, the nurses worked with patients who were single amputees disabled with injury to the remaining leg. The physicians' plans of care identified the patients only as single amputees, omitting other needed information. One patient, for example, was an elderly woman, wheelchair bound, and home alone all day.

In another instance (Case 11), a man facing a second amputation had just become engaged to be married and saw the loss of his leg as the potential loss of his fiancée as well. In that case adaptive care was aimed at helping all members of this family understand how independence and vitality could be preserved even with a second amputation. This was done by counseling as well as physically ''walking through'' all of his valued activities in the house and seeing how they could be managed if he were a double amputee.

In nine cases there were multiple patients in the home. In the Lamarski household (Case 17), all three sisters had disabilities and the two caregiver sisters experienced crisis illnesses (chest pains and retinal detachments) during the care of their sister. The nurse adapted care to assist all three with their disabilities. In an instance in which three patients in one household all required daily dressings, the nurse visited more often than might be considered necessary for just one patient and helped deliver care for each one. She explained the extra visits and the extra care this way:

''I think of the family as a resource and it's my job to preserve it. This lady has to do dressings on her mother and on her father and on her husband. She had to give up her job to do this. I feel I can give her support to make her job easier.''

One patient, Mr. Navarrone (Case 14), required continuous custodial care and was being maintained at home by his daughter and son-in-law. His daughter's post-mastectomy problems made it difficult for her to provide continuous care for her father. The nurse was able to devise ways of lifting and turning the patient that decreased the burden on the daughter.

In two other cases the patient was the most stable person in the household and was caring for even more debilitated members. One of these was a man recovering from surgery whose wife was mentally incompetent and followed him quietly wherever he walked throughout the house (Case 24, Chapter 6). He cooked for her, fed her, and saw to her safety. The nurse was able to obtain a home health aide so the husband could have time to rest and recuperate but who actually was for care of the wife. In yet another case (Case 13), the main caregiver was an unreliable alcoholic woman and the nurse gave her counseling and referral and provided a way to follow up on care she gave the primary patient.

The study showed that at times care was being attempted where resources were so inadequate that the patient's safety would have been sorely compromised without creative and committed adaptation by the nurse. A good example is Mrs. Maclure (Case 15), the woman still desperately ill following excision of clavicle and ribs from osteomyelitis. She had no heat, no medications, and no reliable regular caregiver. The nurse arranged for all three and in addition devised safe and efficient ways to care for the patient's wounds, to ambulate her, and to assure proper nutrition. Another example is the bedridden Mrs. Drago (Case 7), who is alone 16 hours a day. Although the nurse provided extra, ''free'' visits to assure as much continuity and safety as possible, this woman still was in jeopardy and the care regime still was being modified at the time of the observed visit.

In 26 cases, the nurses adapted care ordered in the home to meet the special needs of the patient or the family. In seven of those cases, the physicians' plans of care gave some indication of the special circumstances that might impinge on the services ordered; in the remaining 19, the nurses identified those factors. The additional information needed for home adaptation did not qualify a plan as inadequate unless data for minimum needed skilled care were missing.

The final case study is of the only patient who was ineligible for care by all three criteria: he was not homebound, was not receiving skilled care, and did not have a physician's plan of care.

Case 22: Carmine Fresni

Carmine Fresni, who is 69 years old, was discharged recently from the hospital with a colostomy as the result of cancer metastasis. He previously had had an ileoconduit and cares for that superbly well. He is immaculate and demanding about his personal hygiene. The colostomy has posed no problems and he has assumed the care as though he had always had such a routine.

He is living with his daughter and her family but is ill at ease in the small house with two teenagers and is very eager to get back to his own apartment and his own friends. Because there are 86 steps up to his apartment, he has not yet been able to move back but his remaining minor weaknesses have not kept him from getting out of the house.

The morning of our visit he had spent three hours with a friend at the local shopping mall and had enjoyed a hot dog at Nathan's Famous. When he shares this with his nurse she says with a grin, ''Let's not tell Medicare about your travels'' and Mr. Fresni smiles conspiratorily. The nurse also discusses with him his future concerns about new metastases, the care they will cause, and whether he will be able to stay ''clean'' and ''not smell.''

The patient's referral portion of the physician's plan of care for Mr. Fresni is filled in but it is not a plan, but simply descriptions:

1. rectal tumor between scrotal area and rectum that will eventually eat through his skin
2. uses Chux to catch seepage
3. basically independent, needs reassurance
4. regular diet—appetite good
5. Tylenol q 4 hours

"Needs reassurance" is the closest this comes to being a plan but nothing is known about Mr. Fresni's needs for assurance. Is he aware of his prognosis? What does he need reassurance about? It might be thought from the physician's plan that Mr. Fresni is a man with inoperable cancer waiting for the disease to "eat through his skin."

In fact he has had multiple surgeries already, with an ileoconduit and colostomy. Nothing on his referral form, not even the diagnosis section, gives any hint that he has had a colostomy, yet that is the reason for his care eligibility. He is not using Tylenol but is relying on a mixture of morphine and Dexedrene that appears nowhere on the physician's plan.

The nurse's care was aimed at the areas of Mr. Fresni's real and important concerns. She assured him of her continued interest and availability when he needs it, and both knew that those times were in the near future. She reviewed with him his colostomy care and his sleep pattern. He is requiring more pain medication and is worried that the resulting sleepiness will impinge on his outings with his friends. He worries that he may never be able to return to his own apartment because of all the stairs he must climb and they discuss the possibility of a different apartment, but one in his own neighborhood. The nurse has initiated inquiries regarding such an apartment since Mr. Fresni's daughter does not think he should live alone and is unwilling to assist with plans for him to move.

The nurse also is helping Mr. Fresni to follow a diet to obtain optimum nutrition in spite of his ileoconduit and colostomy. Both have a good laugh over his hot dog lunch. Perhaps the most important nursing service, however, is counseling—assurances that someone is helping him with adequate pain relief and that he will have support in achieving independent living again—and the opportunity to talk with someone about his continuing fears and problems. The nurse is the only person he wants to share these concerns with and her supportive exchange is very therapeutic. When we leave she tells me, "I'd probably move in with him if I had to to keep him going."

Inadequate plans were written more often by specialist physicians than by primary care doctors. The implications of this finding are serious. The study agency reported that an increasing percentage of its Medicare population was being seen for trauma care. The patients in the study group who were trauma patients most often were seen by surgeons, who also ordered their home care. If the population being seen by specialist physicians should increase, so would the number of inadequate plans.

Further analysis of the inadequate plans showed that the least likely deficiency was treatment for the immediate medical problem and the most likely was inadequately identified or planned care for the underlying condition or for secondary diagnoses. The implications of this finding also are serious. The elderly tend to have multiple conditions, and most of those over 65 have at least one chronic disease. The care for those diseases tends to be overlooked when an acute episode of illness occurs.

As the elderly population grows and its members live longer, the number of patients with secondary diagnoses also will increase. As they become patients on home service for a crisis episode, care for their other long-standing conditions may be omitted. Care requirements for chronic disease often change in response to another unrelated crisis episode.

The two most common chronic conditions identified in the study population were diabetes and arteriosclerotic heart disease. Most of the skilled care needs omitted in physician plans and identified by nurses were for secondary diagnoses—most commonly the "forgotten" care of hypertension and diabetes. Both conditions require changes in therapy and in monitoring when any health crisis episode occurs; blood pressure and cardiac output may fluctuate, and insulin or diet changes may be needed. Omission of these observations may compromise the return to health of the individual being treated. Most members of the Medicare population require a comprehensive plan of care during treatment of an episode of illness.

For all 25 inadequate plans, the missing needed information was obtained by the nurse on the initial assessment visit. Federal efforts to lower costs of home health services directly influence the future capability of obtaining that important information. Cost caps on Medicare home health visits—the maximum levels set for reimbursement to be paid by the government for each visit—limit the repayment allowed. Cutting cost per visit means either reducing the length of the visit so that more can be made per day, or using a lower salaried caregiver to provide the service. If either of these strategies is implemented there is less likelihood that comprehensive information for an adequate plan will be obtained.

Public health nurses can and do seek out that necessary information, as has been shown in the data from this study. However, they are the most highly salaried personnel providing home health nursing services and require time to obtain information and implement an effective plan. Cost caps, by decreasing the amount of reimbursement per visit, will force the nurses to make more visits per day (in order to bring in the same revenue per day), and more visits a day means less time per visit. Therefore, visits in the future may be limited to tasks ordered on the physician's plan of care, with the "extra" data gathering being lost.

LOWER LEVEL PERSONNEL: A SOLUTION?

The other strategy to live within reimbursement restrictions is for home health services agencies to use less highly trained personnel to make home visits, thereby decreasing costs per visit. If this strategy is used, public health nurses, who are expert in obtaining comprehensive information and in devising effective plans, will not be used as often to provide these services to patients. Whether or not less professional caregivers can obtain the same needed data and give the same high-quality care is yet to be seen.

If not, and only implementation of an existing physician's plan of care is accomplished, the letter of the law, but not its intent, will have been accomplished. The letter of the law states that only skilled care, directed by a physician, will be reimbursed. The intent of the law, however, is to achieve cost-effective convalescence after an acute illness. Even when a plan is considered adequate and technically easy to carry out, the effectiveness of the visit would be compromised without professional nursing intervention.

For example, Ellen Lamarski (Case 17) required decubiti care and cardiopulmonary monitoring. Those tasks, when provided by the nurse, required very little beyond what the physician ordered and that plan was considered adequate. The reality of a visit to that household, however, showed that far more sophisticated intervention was necessary than simply skilled care. All three sisters required help for themselves and assistance in giving each other care. They also needed continuing support in their mission to maintain Ellen at home.

Although the plans deemed inadequate were judged only on the basis of directing minimal needed skilled care, far more were deemed wanting if the complex services required were to be given effectively. The nurses in the cases studied:

- took extensive family health histories
- made home safety assessments
- reviewed medications
- adapted care to the home setting

- included family members in the care treatment
- contacted community agencies to provide additional needed services
- coordinated medical appointments
- provided counseling, teaching, and home health maintenance care necessary to the patients.

None of these services are reimbursed by Medicare. Medicare patients are benefiting from such "extra" services and from the medical care planning done by the nurse that was omitted by the physician. In most instances the nurses' identification of the extra skilled care needed may have saved Medicare money:

- The extra skilled needs so identified were, by definition, necessary to the resolution of the illness under treatment. Therefore, without that information, care could have been less effective and perhaps longer and costlier.
- No new patients were identified for service in this way; only those already admitted to service had these extra skilled needs pinpointed.

Data from this study show that recovery from an acute episode depends in part on adequate continuing treatment for chronic conditions and that preventive and maintenance services often are necessary complements to skilled care. Some of that necessary care involves the support provided by families (and by nurses in the absence of families) and can be critical to a patient's recovery.

In the study population, professional nursing services such as teaching, counseling, and health maintenance were provided to all but one of the 50 patients. These services, although nonreimbursable, were beneficial either in preventing institutionalization or in strengthening patients' existing health.

Medicare reimburses medically directed care by nurses in the home to patients as an alternative to their institutionalization during convalescence from an acute episode of illness. This study shows that Medicare actually is paying for a far different complement of services. Preventive and maintenance care were provided to all but one of the patients but needed skilled service to only slightly more than two-thirds of the patients.

The needs of patients recuperating at home are nursing, not medical. Having that care directed by a physician is artificial, expensive, and unproductive. It has been widely recognized that tertiary or nursing (not medical) diagnoses are predictors of home care needs, and it is services needed, not medical conditions, that determine such costs (Kurowski, 1979; HSA, 1977; Omaha VNA, 1980).

Physicians are expert in the diagnosis and treatment of illness, but once patients enter convalescence their needs are greatly influenced by their self-care abilities, support systems, home environment, and personal beliefs about what they should be doing to get well. All of these factors have little to do with the medical care provided by physicians to acutely ill persons in an institution or an office. The success of care in those settings generally relies more on physicians' skill than on the patients' self-help abilities or family supports.

Convalescence is a very different process. Here success depends greatly on patients' self-care abilities and on their physical and social environment. This requires the work of a professional to assess that situation and plan care that uses the strengths and makes up for the weaknesses in each situation. This professional is most useful when working in that environment, attuned to the interactions of patient, family, and environment, and skilled in developing successful therapy and goal achievement within that matrix. That professional is not the physician (who the statute charges with home care direction) but the nurse.

Although physicians nominally direct home care, determinations essentially are made by the nurses with great functional autonomy, as noted earlier. Physicians, more out of faith than knowledge, believe that the care they order is the care needed and the care subsequently given. Because nurses do have functional autonomy, care provided in the home tends to be more comprehensive and need-oriented than purely episodic and convalescent.

One of nurses' concerns is how to justify minimum eligibility criteria in order to give care they see as needed; to do so, they tend to rely on literal interpretation of the statute and regulations. The statute requires homebound and skilled care status to be certified by the physician, not the nurse, and both criteria are based on the existing medical condition. If a patient operationally is not homebound, or is receiving primarily nonreimbursable professional services, the letter of the law still is being met. Homebound status is based on the medical diagnoses and on patients' functional capabilities and does not require documentation to justify that categorization.

In the interpretation of skilled care eligibility, nurses were careful never to lie about a skilled need but they may have embossed the little evidence they sometimes had to legitimatize needed services.

As for the third policy, medical plan of care, nurses regularly write the plans for the physicians to sign. Clearly, the physicians are not developing the operational plans, although the statute and regulations continue to read as though that were happening. The nurses are not manipulating this policy, the intermediary is playing ostrich.

A different problem occurs when the patient's status or needs are understated. This is demonstrated by the seven patients who were so severely disabled or ill they could have qualified for institutionalization. The question arises whether the policy should have a maximum level of dependency beyond which home care no longer is appropriate and therefore no longer reimbursable or whether, instead, a different kind of home care services should be allowable.

This is a serious ethical problem, for to deny home care services to the severely disabled is to leave them on their own or force them into institutions. Patients' fear of nursing homes was apparent even in the elderly who were not candidates for immediate placement there. For instance, Mr. Mendota (Case 11), who feared being relegated to a wheelchair as a double amputee, talked about his ultimate idea of tragedy: having to enter a nursing home. For those who were candidates, they or their families all spoke unhappily of that possibility during the visit observed. Ann Lamarski said more than once during our visit to her bedridden sister Ellen (Case 17), "I promised her—never a nursing home." Mrs. Drago (Case 7), the bedridden woman who lived alone, spent most of the visit whispering to her nurse to be assured again and again that the researcher was not really a nursing home placement person in disguise.

ON THE HORNS OF A DILEMMA

With home care service delivery as it is now, the decision about where to give care to the severely disabled elderly is not easy. What may preserve physical safety (institutionalization) may not preserve mental or emotional well-being. Nurses have a responsibility to decide whether patients can utilize care allowed by Medicare. If not, the nurses are expected to deny coverage under Medicare and either place the patients on a self-pay regime or refer them to appropriate care elsewhere.

However, if patients have excessive care needs, the choices are less clear, since placement in a nursing home is one ultimate decision (the other being hospitalization in cases of acute illness). Nurses often opt to keep the patients on home care and give extra unreimbursable service. One nurse related that she regularly saw five "undocumented" patients for such services. Obviously these extra services are not truly "free." When a nurse is providing extra unreimbursable care, the number of reimbursable visits per day obviously must drop; when the number is lower, the cost per visit rises, and the payer of legitimate care therefore expends more in order to cover the costs of those extra services.

All Medicare eligibility policies are manipulated by nurses. Although skilled care is a major eligibility criterion, fewer patients received it than other nonreimbursable professional services and nearly a third of the patients in the study had no need for it. The homebound criterion not only is easily manipulated but actually may increase utilization of Medicare home health services by encouraging those who are permanently homebound to request skilled care. The third policy, requiring a medical plan of care, was nominally followed in the cases studied, but is useless in practice because all 50 plans for patients were rewritten by the nurse following the initial home visit.

The extent of unreimbursable (and therefore unevaluated) care becomes clear when the overall eligibility of the 50 patients is examined (Table 5-10). When the true homebound status is known, the current need for reimbursable care is

Table 5-10 Comparison of Patients Who Met All 3 Eligibility Criteria

	Reimbursable Care	Homebound	Reimbursable and Homebound	Physician Plan of Care	All Three Criteria
Patients Met Criteria	34	31	22	48	22
Patients Did Not Meet Criteria	16	19	5	2	1

determined. The presence of a physician plan of care identified only 22 patients (44 percent of the study population) who met eligibility for Medicare home health services. More than half of the total 50 patients did not meet one or more of those criteria. However, 49 out of 50 were receiving nonreimbursable (and therefore free) services. None of that "extra" care was being evaluated or costed out.

In all three policies, only a physician's certification is needed to initiate service: the physicians certify homebound status and need for skilled care simply by signing their name—no indicators or justifications need be written. The same is true for the physician plan of care: as long as it is signed by the physician, that is sufficient—the content is not examined.

THREE CONCLUSIONS

The factors that influence nursing decisions became apparent from the data for all three policies. Three main themes explained the majority of divergences from policy:

1. Nurses extend nonreimbursable home care services more often to patients who live alone (a) to provide surrogate family care and/or (b) to provide professional teaching and counseling necessitated by the individuals' being alone.
2. Nurses maintain home care services after eligibility lapses when patients are in need of multiple nursing services because the aggregate services are not available elsewhere.
3. Nurses continue patients on home care when their needs require home adaptation. This was a particularly common reason for continuing home care when a patient was not homebound.

All three themes provide overwhelming evidence that nurses maintain patients on home care services in order to give professional nursing care. Teaching and counseling were particularly important for patients who lived alone but it also was apparent that the multitude of nursing services needed by so many, and the home adaptation required for successful self-care, were major factors.

Politically aware of the regulations as well as of the value physicians place on their role as directors of care, nurses understate the authority they have assumed in the delivery of home health services. By mandating one thing (episodic convalescent medical care in the home) and putting physicians in charge of that care, policymakers predict that medical care will result. However, the operational arm of that policy is the public health nurse. The nurse is the only one who sees the patient, who knows the health needs, family, and home situation in a dynamic interaction.

Hospitalized patients and their acute care needs may have very little relevance to convalescent care in the home, as the data in this study demonstrate.

REFERENCES

Home health care: Its utilization, costs, and reimbursement. New York: Health Services Agency of New York City, November 1977.

Kurowski, B. *Cost per episode of home health care: Executive summary.* Boulder, Colo.: University of Colorado, Center for Health Services Research, March 1979.

Mundinger, M.O. *The relationship between policy and practice in the delivery of Medicare home health services* (Doctoral dissertation, Columbia University, 1981).

Omaha Visiting Nurse Association. *A classification system for client problems in community health nursing.* Department of Health and Human Services, HCFA. Washington, D.C.: U.S. Government Printing Office, 1980.

Chapter 6

Public Health Nursing: Little Red Riding Hood Revisited

Public health nursing has changed greatly since the onset of Medicare and the subsequent development of home health agencies. Public health nurses must have a baccalaureate degree—this is the only field of clinical nursing that requires a college-based education. Public health nurses generally are professionals who value flexibility and self-direction in their work, and indeed the community setting requires those personal attributes.

The establishment of Medicare brought an acute care medical focus to public health nursing and has been imposing improved efficiency standards on home care of patients. More and more agencies are looking for nurses with nurse practitioner training because physical assessment and disease management skills increasingly are needed in home nursing. More patients are being discharged before their medical conditions are well stabilized, which requires competent nursing assessment and therapy at home by nurses.

The research study in Chapter 5 was designed to include only public health nurses. Registered nurses without college preparation are employed in the community setting but not as public health nurses and therefore not as the primary caregivers. The nurses observed (all women in this agency) ranged from one working in her first job after college to an older woman, near retirement age who only recently had returned to school to obtain her baccalaureate degree. They had very different backgrounds in nursing, from an Irish nun working in a rural parish hospital to a Hispanic woman working with derelicts in an urban ghetto. However, they brought some of the same perspectives and goals with them to the care of the elderly in this suburban township. Those similarities included a global perspective about needs of the family, not just the patient, and inquisitive problem-solving minds that precluded giving up on any concern they had for patient welfare, an assertive attitude, and political savvy.

Nurses in the agency where patient visits were observed readily discussed with the author why they practiced in the public health field. Some of their comments follow:

"I guess when I worked in the hospital it bothered me that we made other people too dependent. Every day someone different would come in and pull these people out of bed and send them somewhere, and the next day someone new would come and do it a different way. No one would take the time to see if they could do it themselves without help. I guess I wanted to work with people in a setting where I could have more influence in helping them in ways that I felt more comfortable with."

*   *   *   *   *

"In the morning when I'm planning my care I'll usually call the old people I'm going to visit. They worry that you're not coming or they won't be ready if they have to have things ready for me. We interrupt their privacy and their structure. They want us to do what we have to, but then. . . ."

*   *   *   *   *

"When I hire a nurse I look for her affinity for older people, maybe a story in her past, or life experiences. Usually a nurse will tell you she didn't have enough time in the hospital to do teaching or counseling and she usually is a nurse who sees the family as the focus of care. I look for someone who has the ability to be organized within a setting that is disorganized." (Supervisor)

*   *   *   *   *

"Public health nursing attracts a different kind of nurse, one who really likes to be independent and do things with flexibility. This means you have to share and help out because no one can do everything all the time and you only have each other to turn to."

*   *   *   *   *

"I have six kids, three dogs, two cats, and a cranky husband . . . do I think of myself as a woman? No, I always think of myself as a nurse. If someone asked me what I do, I'd say I'm a nurse. I love my work. I am one of the few people who can walk away from their job at the end of a day and say I did something that no one else can do for that guy.'' (This was Kathleen, the subject of the day-long observation described later in this chapter.)

* * * * *

''Time with people in the hospital is so superficial. You see more needs in the patient's home, and your authority is higher there. I am finding it very exciting learning to trust my own judgment again.''

Nurses in the agency were very aware of the family and home settings that are so much a part of their care. They saw the family as a resource to be respected and to be conserved. Whenever they gave care that was being provided at other times by family members, they justified the visit as resource-supportive. They also saw it as an opportunity to assess changes and to teach the family. The nurses also recognized conflicts in families and sought to remedy them. Some of the following statements demonstrate their family awareness:

''People don't understand that families need support. You can't omit aide service just because there is family available. That resource has to be protected.''

* * * * *

''When the family needs support in order to give care, I think that is important for me to do. It's good to know what networks people have, who does what for whom. . .''

* * * * *

''Nurses are intimately part of families in public health. Part of the privilege and part of the responsibility they feel is from that intimacy.'' (Supervisor)

* * * * *

''I see the symbiosis in these visits . . . very few are doing a labor of love or even commitment. Sickness destroys families.''

Nurses also provided care to family members of patients, although they were not considered part of their caseload, nor were the visits billed as extra services. In more than one instance blood pressures were taken, diets were modified, and medications were explained for other family members. In one household all three members were receiving nursing care and health supervision but only one was being carried as the patient. When questioned about these ''free'' activities, the nurses said the added paperwork prevented them from opening these cases as separate visits.

Nurses scheduled regular visits to their patients but found that their planned week always was disrupted. The nurses observed in the study regularly planned more visits than they were able to accomplish; new admissions, or calls for added assistance from patients, added to their schedules.

Only once during the 24 days of observation did the nurses being observed stop for lunch. Often they were returning to the office to begin charting after 4 o'clock, when their workday should have ended. It was highly unlikely that they were giving care to ineligible patients in order to fill idle nursing time—they didn't have any. The administrator discussed plans for expansion in the agency, both physical space and added professional personnel, to meet increased demands for services.

Supervisors assigned new patients but the nurses themselves decided which visits could be omitted, replanned, or traded on any given day. An overriding priority in these determinations was to maintain a sense of continuity with their patients. This was how one nurse explained it:

> ''What happens is you *have* to see the patient who is scheduled for three times a week. The care is too acute to wait. So the once-a-week patients get shoved to the next day or taken over by your back-up. When you miss a whole week of seeing someone you really lose continuity. Usually you are teaching them something, and the other nurse can't go on to the next step like you can. Sometimes you lose primary patients by letting someone else see them, and they are the ones who used to be your everyday visits. It's important to see them through, to see them finally ready to be discharged from home care.''

Patients most likely to be seen by more than one nurse during their home care tenure were those with conditions requiring daily care or those who presented problem conditions that could benefit from the knowledge and creativity of many nurses. One of the truly professional aspects of care in the agency was the openness the nurses showed to each other regarding suggestions for care. This was further enhanced by their behavior during visits from other nurses. They quickly acquainted themselves with care needed and were careful to follow and commend the primary nurse's plan with the patients. Only in the privacy of communication with the primary nurse were alternative suggestions made.

Three incidents in particular demonstrated this collegial atmosphere. On a Saturday, when all visits were made by a nurse who had no permanent caseload and who therefore knew none of the patients, a man with chronic lung disease was seen who clearly had developed new symptoms suggesting the onset of pneumonia. The nurse not only contacted the physician but first called the primary nurse to help assess the change. In the second case, a nurse filling in for a sick colleague found that a patient with end stage renal disease was experiencing increased blood loss and again phoned her nurse colleague to discuss the change before calling the physician. In the third case, a patient being seen for a leg ulcer dressing obviously was healed but the interim nurse delayed discharge until her colleague returned from a one-day holiday.

On other occasions nurses phoned into the agency office for advice on an unanticipated problem, and one of the supervisors there was always able to come up with a suitable idea. Sometimes the supervisor would leave the office and meet the nurse at the patient's home and they would work out the problem together.

Nurses observed in this study liked their work, and planned to stay. One said: "When I found this job I thought I'd found heaven. That was four years ago and I still feel that way." However, they all related factors that posed real problems. Many talked of those problems as the reasons for burnout or loss of optimism and energy to carry on in their work. Their comments helped to tell that story.

"Burnout is faster in public health nursing. In the hospital you can always just pick up the phone and call social service with a problem, or when 3 o'clock comes you just go home and someone else takes over. Also, the emotional load is heavier here. Every single aspect of life is something you're involved with with these people. You're the last link with them, their last hope to remain at home and function as human beings . . . as citizens. And there's the frustration of dead-end hopes of patients. They're dumped with you because no one else can do anything for them. Like a diabetic patient I have who is slowly getting gangrene. I go in and care for his feet. I know he's going to lose them but he's always hopeful. He'll say, 'If only I could get my feet going I'd be OK' and I have to hear those hopes everytime I go in and it's hard."

*   *   *   *   *

"My biggest problem is working within the confines of Medicare. Like I have a terminal cardiac patient who is slowly getting worse. He doesn't need skilled care but if *I* go, all his support care goes—the aides, the hospital bed. That's hard for me to live with."

*   *   *   *   *

"I think nurses are just getting to realize that Medicare is not the law of the land but just another insurance company."

*   *   *   *   *

"We have to accept Medicare as just another health insurance policy, not socialized med. You have to understand that they are not going to pay for everything."

*   *   *   *   *

"Sometimes the responsibility is awesome. We take on more than we can do. You feel such a responsibility for patients. They share things with you that no one else knows . . . when they sleep . . . when they shit . . . how much money they make . . . what they're afraid of. And they depend on you and rely on you for everything."

*   *   *   *   *

"It's hard for me to really accept that people have problems I can't solve. People rely on us for everything, like getting an oil delivery when they have no money. Not only do they feel helpless, I feel helpless as well."

*   *   *   *   *

"The biggest problem here is the whole contradiction in Medicare. The supervisors are thoroughly brainwashed. The staff people are made to feel they are meeting their own needs when they go beyond the skilled guidelines. They reinforce the Little Red Riding Hood image . . . going out to save grandmother. It's a safe role to play, but then the supervisor comes in in the mother role and says Medicare won't pay for it. Lots of staff become very emotionally upset by this contradiction . . . they cry. So many people go into nursing because they want to save people and this conflict leads to the situation where nurses complain about their virtues. They'll say, 'Oh I'll never learn, I'm still teaching Mr. So & So even though I know Medicare won't pay.' "

*   *   *   *   *

"Burnout usually happens because they try to do too much. Part of it is the rescue fantasy . . . they hope they can solve all the problems. Burnout happens to supervisors, too. It usually shows up when I just can't listen anymore. Instead of helping people make decisions, you start giving them the answers, telling them what to do. Sometimes that is appropriate, but usually the best thing is to help them see for themselves what to do.'' (Supervisor)

*   *   *   *   *

''One of the problems for nurses in this agency is that they are supposed to be coordinators of care and yet the services they are supposed to coordinate aren't available. For instance, physical therapy is contracted for on a fee-for-service basis. That means physiotherapists aren't available for conferences or joint planning. Some health agencies contract with us for nursing service—they are the ones that are in contact with the doctor, and therefore there is no communication between our nurses who give the care and the doctor who is ordering the care.'' (Supervisor)

*   *   *   *   *

''I couldn't do this work five days a week. There are just too many people on their last legs.'' (Weekend Nurse)

Nurses in this study had routines that were predictable for each day and yet the problem solving and decision making that went into such a day were incredibly unpredictable. Following is an account of one of the observation days.

A DAY IN THE TRENCHES

It is Friday the 16th of January. The month has been one of the coldest in memory, and each day has been brilliant and icy and bitter cold. Today it is again near zero. When I arrive at the agency at 8 o'clock, I check in with the supervisor to see which nurse I have been assigned to. Nurses have been telling me ''go out with Kathleen, you'll learn a lot about what we do'' and today I learn that I will have that opportunity. Kathleen is about 40, looks younger, has shoulder-length, reddish-brown hair, a happy and attractive face, and a friendly, breezy, self-assured manner.

She is relaxed and professional in her early morning conversation with her care group. Like most of the nurses, she has a small stack of reference books on her desk and uses them this morning to finish the specific plan of care she is formulating for a new admission. She speaks of her patients as though they belong to her. She makes such comments as, ''I'm getting him ready to go home to his sister's house,'' or ''I'm mostly going in today to make sure he's ready for the weekend.'' She makes some telephone calls—one to a patient telling him when she'll arrive and one to give instructions to the aide for a patient from whom she needed a urine specimen.

Kathleen's care group consists of four nurses. They banter among themselves about problem patients or problem doctors. They also consult each other about ways to go about their work in the care they are planning. Most have a cup of coffee while planning their day.

There are about 30 nurses in this office on the fifth floor of a high-rise office building. They sit at their desks in groups of two or four in the large, carpeted room, with window-walls overlooking the parkway. One wall is lined with telephone cubicles and the phones are busy constantly during the first hour or so after the office opens. Some of the nurses are talking in English or Spanish with their patients, some are arranging delivery of equipment or supplies, and some are conferring with physicians. These nurses are quiet, busy, attentive to each other and the milieu in the office is happy for the most part.

One supervisor, who seems to be more directive than the others, is being quietly but firmly ignored by the nurses she is supposed to be supervising. The nurses nod to her suggestions but seem to be planning their care in ways that are unresponsive to her ideas. For instance, "You're not going to visit the Smiths twice this week are you? He's really much better." "Well, yes, he is. Mrs. Smith's the problem," and the Smiths' card goes in the day's pile of planned visits.

The nurses are universally attractive—perhaps because they seem to have such pride and self-assurance in what they are doing. Navy blue is the dress code for public health nurses, and the coat rack is a mass of long navy coats. Blue uniforms are in the minority, with most nurses wearing navy slacks or navy wool skirts, blazers, or sweaters, and white blouses. They do not look like uniforms but they signal the public, especially in unsafe areas, that this is a visiting nurse at work.

Although Kathleen seems relaxed about her preparation, and talks with a number of nurses about patients, she is the first one to leave the office. She has planned her day so that the first visit is to a man whose wife is becoming impatient with his care. The second will be to a woman she had seen just the day before but who was so ill that Kathleen is eager to check on her. The third call will be on one of her favorites, a retired policeman, an Irishman who is receiving long-term care. Last she will visit an elderly bedridden lady who may have a urinary tract infection, and Kathleen wants to take a urine specimen to the lab.

Travel time between patients is a factor in the planning, too. The nurses leave their final travel plans, including telephone numbers of patients to be visited, with the office secretary. They call this "leaving my trail." If calls come in during the day from patients who need to be seen, the primary nurse can be reached and possibly make that extra visit, or at least a phone call.

It has begun to snow. Small flakes are falling steadily as we leave the office and head down the parkway at 9 o'clock. Kathleen's car has sand in the trunk, flashlights, a flare, and a jack, as well as her black bag packed with the standard supplies: dressings, tape, a thermometer, scissors, a Fleet Brand Enema, and sometimes, if needed, a syringe. It is a short drive to Lawrence Walton's apartment house, and she finds a parking place right in front of the building. On our way I have asked: "What are the biggest barriers you find in giving care?" Although we arrive at Mr. Walton's at 9:30, we don't leave the car for nearly half an hour as Kathleen fills me in on what those barriers are.

"I've been a nurse nonstop for 21 years and the longer I work the less use I have for doctors . . . in my Karma I'm sure I'll come back as a doctor. This one man I have still has a T-tube in two months after his surgery. His surgeon, and that's in quotes, just can't be bothered. With another patient's urine, I went to three different labs yesterday and all the labs were closed. That doctor . . . and that's also in quotes . . . when I finally reached him said, 'Well, girlie, I'll just order it again tomorrow.' "

I asked how she responded to "girlie." She said if a patient needed something she would play the game to get what she wanted for that person.

"Communication with doctors is my biggest problem. We're dealing with 'Dr. Schlepheimer' who hasn't opened a book in years. For instance, I've got this man with cancer of the colon who had all kinds of problems in the hospital. He's a real gentleman and it was a long time before he was comfortable telling me this. It seems that the day after his surgery he is still groggy and he wakes up and tells me this guy is at the foot of his bed and says, 'Hey buddy'—that's how this doctor talks to him— 'Hey buddy, I broke off your front three teeth putting the tube down yesterday.' The man had an MI [myocardial infarction] while he was in the hospital, and after he got home was passing kidney stones. I saw the stones and they were huge yet he hardly complained.

"So when he starts telling me he has slight rectal pain I figure it may be more than slight. His temperature is 99 so I called his doctor and asked him for more information about his hospital picture. I knew he had rectal abscess there and I ask what grew out on the culture and the bastard wouldn't tell me. He said, 'Look honey, don't call me unless his temp is 102 or 101.' I said that with a base line temp of 97 I was concerned with 99 and he said, 'Tell you what, you worry for the both of us.' So I had him force fluids, more sitz baths, had him take ASA and keep off his rectum and it got better. The doctor was right but I needed to know more. It was different when I worked in the city hospital."

"Why?"

"I'm not sure. Partly I think it was because it was a teaching center and doctors are used to answering questions and learning from each other."

"What other problems do you encounter?"

"Medicare. I have a patient who needs radiotherapy three times a week to reduce his spleen and Medicare will pay for transportation only if he needs oxygen or a stretcher and has to have an ambulance . . . otherwise he has to pay his own transportation. He really can't go out in a car so I called the doctor to order oxygen and the doctor said, 'I'd have problems with that.' I guess there are more abuses with Medicaid but Medicare doesn't do enough."

"What do you do about that?"

"Not much. I call the voluntary agencies. Like a man I have with psoriasis . . . I've never seen such bad psoriasis. When he walked, he rustled. His apartment was wall-to-wall skin. He was constantly flaking. The only part of him not involved was his teeth. I got him to his doctor's office one day and he destroyed the office . . . there was skin everywhere.

"He needed treatment in an ultraviolet box and I finally found there was one at a hospital in the city. He needed transportation to get there and also to have access to its really excellent dermatology clinic. I made 17 phone calls in six hours. I called Catholic Charities because he was a daily communicant, I called senior citizens, I called the Red Cross. They told me that his town and the hospital he wanted to go to were in two different counties and their insurance wouldn't cover them for the transportation. I had had it by then and was practically crying. I said, 'What about San Salvador? The Red Cross goes there and this man is an American citizen! What do you mean insurance?'

"His doctor was a nice man and he came to the rescue. We had a conference and decided that the man's admission would be profitable enough for the local hospital to buy a UV machine, and the doctor convinced administration. Of course, the doctor knew that if I got this man to the city he'd lose a patient, so there was something in it for him too. So the man got his treatment at his local hospital and his Medicare reimbursement paid for the UV machine."

We leave the car, take the elevator to the Waltons' apartment. Mrs. Walton answers the door and we can see her husband in the kitchen in his pajamas eating breakfast. He doesn't speak to us. Mrs. Walton says she needs time to go to the bookmobile and that she is tired of caring for her husband. We stay for a few minutes but we were interrupting his breakfast, so Kathleen agrees to come back later so Mrs. Walton can go to the bookmobile. She clearly is agitated by the prospect of a long weekend housebound with her invalid husband. She already had told Kathleen she could not continue to care for him alone and would put him in a nursing home if the work continued to get her down. Kathleen also offers to give him a bath since his wife was tired and a home health aide could not yet be arranged for. This cheered both husband and wife.

In the car Kathleen begins talking again about the frustrations in her work.

> "I'm unable to do what I want to do. It's the system. Like this urine culture, I have to go and get an order, then no lab is open. And the paperwork—if anything would make me quit, it's the paperwork. Otherwise, this is the only job I've had that I think I could stay in and retire from. When we get a new case in the office you'll hear a groan. It isn't that we don't want to see a new face and do something for somebody, it's the paperwork."

After another 20-minute ride on slippery, snow-covered streets we arrive at 10:45 at our second patient, Florence Feiss (Case 18 in Chapter 5).

> Florence Feiss, who is 69 years old, had been hospitalized for two weeks with congestive heart failure. She has been home, and on home care, for six weeks. Her other diagnoses are:
>
> Aortic stenosis
> Postnecrotic cirrhosis with jaundice
> S/P breast cancer (bilateral mastectomy)
>
> She has two physicians, as her referral notes: Dr. W. for medical follow-up and Dr. K, the gastroenterologist who has hospitalized her most recently. Her orders are:
>
> Aldactone 1-2X week
> 90/40-148/80
> Jobst stocking
> Back brace and bed board
> Sk-APAP #3 1-2X week
> Dig. 0.125 mgm od

Zyloprim 300 mgm od
1500 Cal 2 Gm Na diet

On Kathleen's assessment visit she found that Mrs. Feiss had suffered from osteoarthritis for years (which may account for the back brace and bed board) and that the medications orders were confusing: neither physician knew what Sk-APAP #3 was and there were no guidelines for when to give Aldactone. The medical doctor, when called, refused to follow the patient or monitor the previous medication regime since 'she took up with the gastroenterologist.' The gastroenterologist has not accepted or returned any phone calls from the nurse so Mrs. Feiss has been cared for under the vague set of orders from that specialist since hospital discharge.

Kathleen thinks Mrs. Feiss may have cancer metastases, which account for the mental deterioration and jaundice (and even the back pain), or may have further damage from cirrhosis. Completely frustrated by her inability to get the data she needs from either physician, she has been left the task of visiting Mrs. Feiss and making weekly assessments of her health status.

Mr. and Mrs. Feiss live in an old Victorian house set close to similar houses on a residential street lined with maple trees. The entry hall is mahogany and a large sweeping staircase leads to the second floor with a long hall lined by bedroom-dressing room combinations that now are cramped two-room apartments.

Mr. Feiss is standing in the open door of his kitchen as we arrive and Mrs. Feiss is lying huddled in bed in the bedroom-living room. She is moaning and tremorous. The mattress is covered by a single sheet; an old, worn comforter with the stuffing falling out covers her body. Her gray-black hair is matted and dirty, her skin is dry and yellow, and her face is contorted with either pain or anxiety. She repeatedly moans, "Pop, Pop, Pop, please, please," and seems disoriented, although with Kathleen's calm hand on her shoulder the direct questions receive relevant, concise answers:

"Florence, what's wrong?"
"I don't know."
"Do you hurt anywhere?"
"No."
"Have you had any water today?"
"I don't know."

Kathleen takes her vital signs, inspects her skin, and questions her husband. It appears that Mrs. Feiss has remained in bed the past 22 hours, has not eaten, drunk water, or voided, and had a very restless and confused night. Although Kathleen had left explicit directions and her own phone number with Mr. Feiss to call her if his wife did not improve, Mr. Feiss had been unable to mobilize himself for such a decision. Even now he could only look to Kathleen for direction, and when she told him to sit down and have a cup of coffee, that is exactly what he did. The next hour was a series of attempts to get Mrs. Feiss to a hospital.

The following events demonstrate the kinds of work public health nurses find waiting for them in the course of a day's home visits.

11:10 A.M. Kathleen phones the medical doctor, whose nurse takes a message: 'Mrs. Feiss is in prehepatic coma and I'm sending her to the hospital.' The nurse tells Kathleen she will forward the message to the physician, who will be at the hospital.

11:20 A.M. The nurse calls back to say that the physician will admit her to the hospital when she arrives. Kathleen sits down with Mr. Feiss and tells him his wife must go to the hospital. He looks very relieved. She asks him if he has $45 cash, which he will need for the ambulance, and he does. She explains to him that he will receive Medicare reimbursement for 80 percent of it ($36).

11:20 to 11:30 A.M. The following attempts were made to get an ambulance:

Call to AR Ambulance: One-and-a-half-hour wait unless "absolute emergency."

Call to local police emergency number: It rings without answer.

Repeat call to police emergency number: answered after ten rings and Kathleen is informed that she must go to the proprietary companies first because the police are backup only.

Call to AA Ambulance: When the phone is answered Kathleen says, "I need an ambulance" and is immediately put on hold! The call is reanswered within five seconds (but what frantic phoners would wait?) and this company, too, has a one-and-a-half-hour wait unless an "absolute emergency."

Recall to police emergency: The police agree to come.

Kathleen grins at Mr. Feiss and says, "Put your money away, we got the police ambulance and it's free."

11:30 A.M. Kathleen helps Mr. Feiss gather up his wife's few belongings and her medications and tells him he can ride in the ambulance.

11:40 A.M. The police ambulance comes screaming down the street, going the wrong way. It double-parks, blocking the street and bringing all the neighbors to their windows. Four young men, with official-looking big yellow metal boxes, come charging up the stairs. They take Mrs. Feiss's blood pressure and look hopefully at their IV equipment while Kathleen assures them: "It's not that kind of emergency." They look disappointed. The fifth member of the team (obviously a lieutenant, by his cap) tells Kathleen sheepishly that they cannot transport Mrs. Feiss to the hospital because "she isn't sick enough" and that they have to be free for "real emergencies" as the backup transport. Kathleen understands but asks, "What do I do for this lady? She needs medical care now." The lieutenant agrees and calls one of the proprietaries to make Mrs. Feiss the next priority call. The five men then agree to wait to make sure Mrs. Feiss doesn't turn into a "real" emergency before the other ambulance arrives. Meanwhile two police cars have arrived to offer support to the police ambulance. They decide to stay, too.

12:10 P.M. The second ambulance appears, also going the wrong way on this one-way street, also with sirens blaring. It pulls up and parks behind the first ambulance. Two attendants come up and one asks Kathleen, "Are you a nurse?" "Yes," says Kathleen, "I'm a nurse." He looks again at her navy pantsuit and white blouse and says, "I mean an R.N.?" "Yes," says Kathleen, "I'm the real thing. Can we get this lady to the hospital?" The other attendant looks at Mrs. Feiss, lying trembling and moaning in the bed, and says, "I know what she's got . . . Parkinjun's [sic] disease." They use Mrs. Feiss's sheet to lift her onto the stretcher, walking with wet, dirty feet directly on her mattress as they do so. Having been summoned by the police instead of by the nurse, the ambulance does not have to collect money from Mr. Feiss—it seems true emergency transits are free and are determined by the police, not the nurse.

12:15 P.M.   Mrs. Feiss is finally on her way to the hospital, her husband riding in the ambulance with her. Kathleen makes sure the apartment is locked as we leave and remarks: "See what I mean about transportation?"

En route to our next patient, I ask Kathleen how she feels about her working relationship with physicians. She replies: "They're not helpful. This patient we just saw, he never returned my call yesterday. If I knew more about her medical condition, maybe I'd know better how to explain her behavior and how sick she really is."

We arrive at Joseph McNamara's apartment at 12:30. He lives on the second floor of a pleasant, two-story apartment building in a residential section two blocks from downtown. The front door has a buzzer security system with an intercom that enables him to let us into the building. The three-room apartment is well furnished with carpets and clean, comfortable furniture. Both the McNamaras meet us at the door in their pajamas and robes. Mr. McNamara is 80 years old. Two months ago he suffered a cardiac arrest during surgery for a cholecystectomy. He recovered from the heart problem and was sent home but the surgery never was completed. He still has a draining T-tube in place (the reason for the nursing visits) but neither the surgeon nor the heart doctor will make the decision for Mr. McNamara to have his surgery completed. Kathleen has been talking with both physicians to facilitate the necessary collaboration for such a decision.

Mr. McNamara is a twinkly eyed little man with pink cheeks and an Irish brogue. He shuffles into the bedroom, talking with affection and humor with Kathleen. Mrs. McNamara is a little woman, vague and quiet. She doesn't speak at all during the visit and follows her husband about as though obeying his direction. Her robe is inside out and unbuttoned. While Kathleen does Mr. McNamara's dressing, Mrs. McNamara sits in a chair watching and eventually dozes off. Kathleen tells me later that she is continually forgetful and is unsafe to leave alone. Mr. McNamara cares for her and makes sure she has eaten and gets her rest.

Following his hospitalization he was exhausted by this constant responsibility and Kathleen has arranged for a home health aide—ostensibly for Mr. McNamara, but really for his wife. Once Kathleen discharges this patient, the aide service also will stop. Kathleen checks his vital signs, asks when his next physician's visit is, and they talk about their joint plans to "get the doctors moving." She gives him a big hug and tells him she'll see him next visit and we are gone by 12:55.

On the way to the next patient, who lives in the same apartment complex, I ask Kathleen how she decides on her plan for any given individual. "I look first at the physical problem, then the emotional . . . what they need to help them get through this."

We arrive at the apartment of Angeline Drago (Case 7 in Chapter 5) at 1 o'clock. She is tiny, white-haired, 83 years old, and confined to her bed. She has been receiving home care services for two months following a four-month hospitalization. She has lived alone for years and her hospitalization was necessary after her nieces found her ill and dehydrated. In the hospital she was treated for dehydration, long-standing hypertension, and Parkinson's disease, and a urinary tract infection. She was discharged home with the understanding that her nieces would arrange for 24-hour homemaker service (it is even written in the discharge orders).

Because she is too weak to get out of bed and because she often is incontinent, Mrs. Drago has a Foley catheter. Her nieces arranged for full homemaker service, but recently decreased it to eight hours a day. The other 16 hours a day Mrs. Drago is alone, bedridden, and unable even to switch on a light or dial the telephone. The Foley catheter and unstable cardiac status justify the nurse visits.

Today Kathleen is obtaining a urine specimen because she thinks Mrs. Drago again has a urinary tract infection. She obtains a specimen and instructs the homemaker on encouraging fluids, especially water and cranberry juice, and we leave by 1:15 P.M.

Kathleen discusses the bigger problem with Mrs. Drago—her day-to-day safety. It seems that the nieces may have stolen Mrs. Drago's money and are being very stingy in the care they are willing to purchase for her. Mrs. Drago is sweet and somewhat naive, but alert and lucid. She insists she will never go to a nursing home and will remain home at all costs.

Kathleen knows that Mrs. Drago's safety and health are at risk in the current situation but her only alternatives are to force institutionalization or go to court to obtain access to funds for more comprehensive homemaker assistance. She has gone to court as a patient's advocate before, and the agency paid her for her time. However, she found it took enormous energy and time to prepare for such an effort and was uncertain that such an approach would benefit Mrs. Drago; she thought it might just accelerate the end of the patient's cherished independence.

We head back to the car and find the snow has thickened, with at least an inch covering the hood and windshield. Kathleen plans to return to Mr. Walton but it is too early for his wife to go to the bookmobile so we park near his apartment building and walk down the hill to a coffee shop. Kathleen is planning to drive into Boston tonight to visit an old friend for the weekend. She will take groceries home for her large family before leaving. She says she really needs to relax and just think of herself once in a while and this weekend will give her that chance. Even though this trip is important to her, she is waiting calmly for the bookmobile so she can give Mrs. Walton a respite and Mr. Walton his care. I find myself thinking I would have given the needed care this morning, Mrs. Walton's pleasure notwithstanding, and been on my way out of this storm by 4 o'clock.

We have a cup of coffee (the closest I've been to lunch since this study began) and Kathleen tells me what it was like growing up in a poor but happy and energetic Irish family. She also tells me about her intense dislike of paperwork: "It's enough to make you quit. Actually there are things we don't do now because it takes paperwork. Take a home health aide—you have to fill in a special form and then write up all the supervisory visits. Sometimes it's just easier to do the work yourself. I'm really a hands-on nurse."

However, she tells me that some paperwork doesn't bother her:

"Like verification for patients. I'm willing to lie for some people if they need the care . . . like the Jacobsens (a woman caring for her bedridden husband). Do you think I'd let Medicare discharge him? I'd go to court and raise my hand and swear to anything for him. If they needed it, I guess I'd move in. That is what Medicare is all about . . . helping people like them. I think health care should be subsidies to families. Then, with that little extra money, they could care for their own. There are problems with Medicare, though. Patients will tell you they're 'entitled' to certain care. Some of them could use other services, though, like homemakers."

The other problem Kathleen talks about is the lack of information on patients:

"We do buckshot nursing. We just don't have all the information we need. We never get lab information on the referral and most doctors can't be bothered giving it to you. Even after the patients are on home care we don't get lab reports. Medicare should demand better referrals to us . . . we could give better care and maybe save them some money."

It is 2:30 and we leave to see Mr. Walton. Mr. Walton has chronic leukemia and is homebound because of his long-standing weakness from that disease. He had been hospitalized recently with a combination of leukemic crisis and diabetic ulcers on an ankle. He had returned home with ulcer care and home health aide services ordered.

When we arrive at their beautifully furnished suburban apartment, he is in his pajamas in the bedroom and Mrs. Walton has her hat and coat on ready to leave for the bookmobile. Kathleen tries to encourage her to stay for "just a few minutes" to observe the way to transfer Mr. Walton into the tub but she will have none of it and rushes out the door.

Kathleen bathes him, shampoos his hair, and takes care of his feet. The ulcers that qualify him for care are healed but she creams his feet and puts cotton socks on. When Mrs. Walton returns at 3:20, Kathleen assures her that there will be a home health aide by Monday, and we leave.

In the car Kathleen smiles ruefully and says, "Now that's home health aide work but they both needed it to make it through the weekend."

It is still snowing when Kathleen and I arrive at the office at 3:45. She has decided to do most of her paperwork Monday morning so she simply fills in the records quickly on care given that day, then makes sure a home health aide is assigned for the Waltons. She tells me she'll be "dropping in" on Mr. Feiss to see how his wife is before work on Monday.

Although this day's activities reflect the perspective and practice of only one nurse, it is representative of public health nursing. It takes a special kind of person to practice in the community and in people's homes. The nurse not only is responsible for implementing a medical plan of care, which is a common nursing role, but also must adapt that care to many different settings and resources. In addition, the priorities of actual care given may change according to conditions in the home that day or according to unforeseen changes in the patient's condition.

These factors require that a nurse in the home setting must be flexible, adaptive, creative, and have observation and judgment abilities to know immediately how to proceed with care. In addition, that nurse may be the patient's only professional contact over a period of weeks or months. Physicians must recertify their plans of care at least every two months but there is no requirement that they ascertain whether the patient's needs have changed or that they actually see the patient. Therefore, the nurse in the home has the additional responsibility, unlike other settings, of assessing the patient's need for medical care.

Another difference is that nurses are responsible for seeing their patients as needed and for assuring that their nursing needs have been planned for between visits. This kind of accountability differs from other nursing settings. Usually nurses are employees, responsible for a work shift. During that time they provide care according to the time available and care requirements—what can't be accomplished then will be done on the next shift by someone else (in an institution) or the next set of office hours (in an ambulatory setting).

Ambulatory care visits usually take place when patients initiate the request for service. They visit the caregiver with specific symptoms or as a follow-up. In home care, patients cannot initiate service—except for the first assessment visit, it is the professional who determines whether the individuals can be seen, for what services, and how often. Whereas patients can be seen in an ambulatory setting for almost any reason they choose, home care has a much more restrictive screening process. This places limitations on access and imposes added responsibility on the nurse: how often the patient should be seen, what care should be provided, and by whom all become elements of nursing decision making.

These service restrictions and broadened professional responsibility have developed because nearly all home care is reimbursed by third party payers who naturally want to limit expenses. Ambulatory care lacks those restrictions because it usually is self-pay. Institutional care has restrictions similar to home service, for the same reasons, but in institutions it is physicians, not nurses, who are decision makers about access.

This global responsibility in home care nursing requires professionals who have the skills and the perspective to determine efficient and useful delivery of services. Many nurses shrink from that kind of accountability. Those who find satisfaction in the autonomy and the excitement of self-direction, however, provide an important resource to home care patients and their families. One of the greatest concerns for these nurses is the contradiction in policy that requires medical direction and then supports sub rosa, nursing management on home health services.

Probably the single most important reason for this problem is that nursing still is widely regarded as a dependent arm of medicine. In this view there is no contradiction in having nurses carry out the medical plan; obviously, that is what nurses do traditionally. There is no acknowledgment of the different perspectives between the two professions; indeed, there is no acknowledgment that there are two separate professions. There also is no acceptance of the fact that the home setting and convalescent state of patients make it almost impossible to provide useful care based on decisions by a professional whose perspective is limited to office and institution and whose expertise is acute illness.

The way that Medicare policy is written denies that any decision making is necessary once the medical plan has been formulated by the physician. This has led to the frustrations that nurses experience in providing home care under existing regulations.

Chapter 7

The Need for Change

The findings from the analyses of three Medicare policies discussed in Chapter 5 provide a good deal of insight into the current home health services program. This study identifies four major findings that have implications for administrators and for policymakers:

1. The impact theory of policy direction does not work.
2. Quality and outcome measurement, important components of publicly funded programs, are missing in Medicare home health care.
3. Demographic and cultural changes will necessitate new policy direction for Medicare home health services.
4. Welfare and health policy cannot be isolated operationally.

THE IMPACT THEORY

On the first finding, the impact theory says that if policy is followed, the result (impact) is predictable. It implies that the specific process assures a given outcome. For instance, in Medicaid, social supports are supplied not because of need but because of entitlement. By meeting the criteria (being sick, old, and poor), individuals are entitled to a homemaker in many states. That is so even if they have available and able family members who could have provided those services. Conversely, to be old and sick, but not poor, means that homemaker services are not available even if their absence could cause expensive institutionalization at public expense.

This differentiation in policy was made with the expectation that the poor were more in need of social supports than those with adequate funds. The outcome, however, often is very different. The failure of the impact theory in policy implementation is well illustrated in *Local Success and Federal Failure* (Clinton,

1979), a sociological look at how federal policy was easily (and legally) manipulated for successful local economic development in a rural southern town.

The author's study of home care services again questions the impact theory. Limiting reimbursement to skilled care has not curtailed the services actually delivered, nor has the homebound constraint been invoked regularly to deny services. The data do show that reimbursement criteria have been more effective in limiting admission to care than they have in containing continuation or content of services. The statute and regulations, as noted earlier, require three-fold physician certification: for homebound status, for the need of skilled care, and for a plan of nursing services. The inherent belief in such a highly regulated framework is that the rules will result in (1) only medically curative care's being delivered, and (2) only those who otherwise would be cared for in an institution for that qualifying illness episode. The real-life impact, however, is far different: the rules result in physicians' documentation for all three criteria but the care actually delivered is substantially different.

Policy always will be manipulated for purposes valued by the implementers. In public policy such tactics have more serious implications because those who pay for care are not those who receive the benefits, so the purchaser has accountability to the payer for predictable results. Recognition of policy manipulation makes the determination of probable impact a very sophisticated process and one that needs to be better developed for Medicare.

QUALITY AND OUTCOME

The study's second important finding is that key components of publicly funded programs—quality and outcome—are missing from the Medicare home health services program. Home care policy has been highly regulated in regard to structure and process—home health agencies are well defined and eligibility and direction of care by physicians are specified. Outcome and quality measurements, however, have been developed inadequately (Feder, 1977; Kingsdale, 1978; Van Dyke & Elliott, 1969; Van Dyke & Brown, 1972). Outcomes are not measured at all and quality evaluation is limited to quarterly meetings in the agency, as mandated in the regulations. At these sessions, a utilization review committee looks at a representative number of charts to determine and improve quality and effectiveness of care. The committee is composed of:

1. a physician from the physician's advisory committee
2. a staff nurse
3. the director of patient services
4. the supervisor of nursing
5. a physical therapist
6. the home health aide supervisor

7. a medical social worker
8. a consumer representative (usually a board member).

The charts are distributed to the committee members so that each reviews an equal number. They are analyzed for:

1. what services were needed
2. what services actually were provided
3. how the needs were met
4. whether the services were integrated
5. what progress was made.

Although these five criteria are commendable, Medicare does not pay for services needed unless they are skilled; it also does not require progress measurement or goal achievement. Therefore, for a chart to reflect high-quality care, services that are not reimbursable must be provided. When that quality of care is given, both time per visit and cost per visit rise. At the same time Medicare, concerned with rising costs, has placed increasingly restrictive cost caps on reimbursement levels. It thus is clear that quality is not linked with reimbursement in the Medicare structure and is not promoted by its payment policies.

The author participated in one of the study agency's quarterly Utilization Review Committee meetings. The panel searched diligently in the record and engaged in thoughtful discussions to find ways to improve care in the agency. It reviewed 13 charts. In seven of them, inadequate medical information was the primary deficit (although a smaller sample, 13 as compared to 50 in the author's larger study, this separate population of patients and independent reviewers duplicated the findings in the larger study that 50 percent of physician care plans were inadequate). In the six other charts there was no indication of patient progress. These were the two major findings in the quality assessment, yet neither one is required under Medicare.

Claims Payment System a Key Factor

When Medicare was developed, political necessity and administrative convenience led to the adoption of claims payment through the existing Social Security Administration (SSA), primarily because that agency was deemed large enough to be able to do the job, and local intermediaries for initial claims screening, most notably Blue Cross and Blue Shield, were fully acceptable to physicians and hospitals. However, both of these choices tended to obscure any attempts at quality assessment. Feder (1977) shows how the claims payment system functions: if patients were eligible, the checks were disbursed—no services were entailed, so quality of care in effect was irrelevant. That concept pervaded Medicare's takeover of claims processing: eligibility of the patient still was the key to payment to the institution. No questions were asked concerning the services; information as to appropriateness or quality of care or outcome achieved was not needed for payment. Feder also notes that an overriding need in Medicare was to provide patients with sufficient access to services, so assuring availability took precedence over assuring quality.

The use of Blue Cross and Blue Shield as intermediaries was another factor in the lack of quality assessment. Van Dyke and Elliot (1969) point out that Blue Cross and Blue Shield from their inception were designed to insure institutions against losses from patients' nonpayment. From their beginning in 1929, Blue Cross and Blue Shield have had a two-fold relationship in the insurance industry:

1. risk sharing with subscribers
2. income protecting for hospitals.

In Medicare, the intermediary bears no risk when costs exceed premiums paid, so there is the question of the propriety of giving them stewardship of public funds. Smith and Hollander (1973) raise the same questions in commenting that the desire for operational readiness precluded the timely development of a mechanism to assure accountability to the public for expenditures. Blue Cross and Blue Shield can be more liberal in approving payment to agencies (and insuring their income) when they face none of the risk of excess payment. Therefore, there is no reason to expect such intermediaries to adopt quality controls. Similarly, Medicare home care services do not require any copayment by patients, so they are not involved in direct payment for their services, and thus are less concerned with quality.

The Outcome Assessment Gap

Outcome measurement is the other missing component in Medicare home care policy. There is no way to assess effectiveness of care without measuring the results and without such an evaluation it is difficult to choose between alternate methods of delivering care. For example, the outcomes of comprehensive professional nursing care (what was delivered, in this study) may be very different from the results of providing only medically assistive, curative care (what is reimbursed under Medicare).

Assessment of outcomes has been defined by Donabedian (1969): "Assessment of outcomes is the evaluation of end results in terms of health and satisfaction. It is assumed that good results are brought about, at least to a significant degree, by good care." He also compares outcome measurement with process evaluation:

> Those who focus on process point out their responsibility is to see to it that "the best" medical care, as defined by health experts, is provided. They do not consider it their primary concern to evaluate the effectiveness of the health sciences. By contrast, those who would focus on

outcomes or end results emphasize primary concern for health and for the responsibility of the administration to investigate the causes of failure to achieve health objectives and to take appropriate action.

At this point in the Medicare program, the outcomes of nursing care are inferred to be the results of reimbursable nursing care, yet the data from this study indicate that the two are very different. Given this inference, any outcome measurement attempted would be invalid.

Weissert, a researcher for the National Center of Health Services Research (NCHSR), has conducted a cost-effectiveness study (1980) for the Health Care Financing Administration (HCFA) to determine the advisability of offering supportive home health services under Medicare.

A federal study to cost out the added use of homemakers for Medicare beneficiaries (Weissert, 1979) demonstrates that this service increases satisfaction and decreases mortality, but at a high cost: those who receive homemakers use more services (including institutionalization) and have 60 percent higher costs for care. Others also have conducted cost or patient outcome studies (Berkman & Syme, 1979; Kurowski, 1979) but little has been done to link results with actual content of service. Berkman and Syme found that the elderly who maintain their social ties in their normal environments live longer. Kurowski compared costs of an episode of home care in two different agencies serving two different populations with differing resources.

Outcome measurement in home health services is at the beginning stage of formulation. The research has been extensive but ambiguous. It has been shown that home health services can decrease hospital length of stay (LaVor & Callender, 1976), that they may prevent hospital admissions (Gary, 1979), and that they can decrease overall costs for an episode of illness (Brickner, 1975; Denver VNA, 1976). In contrast, Pegels (1980) reports that expanding the availability of home health services may increase their use and ultimately push up overall health care costs rather than decreasing them through substitution of home services for institutionalization. An overview of cost studies (Hammond, 1979) also shows that increasing home health care as now defined may not decrease institutionalization.

A federal study to estimate the costs of liberalizing eligibility says that each added benefit would increase overall Medicare expenditures.

	Projected Overall Medicare Cost Increase
Eliminating eligibility requirement for skilled care	$1,250,000,000
Eliminating eligibility requirement for homebound status	92,500,000
Adding homemaker services	75,000,000

Another study indicates that the very requirement of skilled care for eligibility may not be cost effective; it may be much more expensive to care for patients who require numerous skilled services (stroke rehabilitation, for instance) at home than in an institution (HCA, 1979). These two studies suggest the problems with the skilled care criterion. The DHEW study suggests that if the skilled care criterion were eliminated, the cost of home care would increase by $1.25 billion a year. This is because eligibility would be open to all the elderly who could use nonskilled support services, such as home health aides. Maintaining the skilled care criterion with no upper limit, however, can lead to home care expenses in excess of what that care would cost in an institution.

Isolation, Not Perspective

All of the cost studies addressed recommended changes as isolated events. For instance, Weissert's (1980) analysis of homemaker assistance was based on the presumption that the rest of the system would remain unchanged and homemakers would simply be an add-on. The same is true of the 1977 DHEW study estimating costs of eliminating the skilled care criterion.

Typical health policy evaluative studies address the components of Medicare home health services without a broader look at the way the system operates and what trade-offs may be useful when changing policy. For example, it may be cost effective to reimburse homemaker assistance under certain limited conditions.

Kate Donnelly required a homemaker (not a nurse or even an aide) to help her dress, shop, cook, and rise from her chair after her accident. Homemaker services following the fracture of her arm could have even prevented her subsequent hospitalization. A homemaker for the Walton family could have provided the assistance needed so that Mrs. Walton might have been willing to assume more of the care of her husband, thereby delaying or preventing his admission to a nursing home. Homemakers are less costly than aides, and family members may be able (and willing) to carry out some of the aide functions if they have the assistance of a homemaker to help with other chores.

Medicare amendments included funds for demonstration developmental research projects to explore changes that can promote cost containment. More of this kind of research must be combined with evaluative studies so that a broader policy perspective can be achieved.

Average length of stay in hospitals has decreased but there is no clear indication that home health care has replaced prolonged hospital stays. Utilization review activities regarding appropriateness of hospitalization may be more responsible for earlier discharges. Home health services to beneficiaries who were not hospitalized account for about a third of the Medicare home health dollars. The data are even less clear as to whether these nonhospital illness episodes would have required hospitalization if home care had not been available. Outcomes other than decreased hospitalization also would be useful in policy evaluation. Health status measurements, for instance, could be used to determine the value of services.

DEMOGRAPHIC AND CULTURAL CHANGES

The third finding in this study is that demographic and cultural changes make new approaches necessary for home health care of the elderly. Home health care planning has been predicated on the theory that professionals deliver the services. Little recognition has been given to the other factors that influence service delivery such as the home setting; available resources; the knowledge, health beliefs, and self-care abilities of the patient; or the availability and assistance of families.

The Family: A Vital Resource

The family resource is a major one and cannot be ignored in the cost and success of home health services. In a study of home health services in New York state, Callahan (1980) estimates that families helped in "significant ways" for 60 to 85 percent of the elderly patients involved. An analysis by Somers (1978) suggests that loss of family, not loss of health, has caused the increased health care costs of the elderly. Davis (1974) notes that increased price, not greater use of services, is the major reason for higher costs. An epidemiological survey of the aged and their mortality (Berkman & Syme, 1979) says that maintenance of social ties for the elderly decrease mortality.

Family assistance is apparent in reimbursable care activities as well as in the custodial and social aspects of care. The data from the author's study show that families can be taught to carry out activities that are reimbursable when done by the nurse (e.g., dressings, irrigations, injections). Other study data show that patients living alone, and therefore without regular family assistance, are kept on service longer, even after eligibility has lapsed.

In the planning of public policy, some attention has been paid to family care. For instance, in the early 1970s, cash subsidies were considered for families that were caring for their elderly members, thus potentially saving public funds that otherwise would have been expended for nursing home care of these individuals. When estimates of the number of eligible families were so high that the plan potentially was very costly, the idea was dropped quietly. However, the concept surfaced again and some surveys showed that "granny funds" or cash disbursements to families would be the most successful method of ensuring their care of the dependent elderly (Callahan, 1980).

This approach surfaced not because public policymakers had any second thoughts about the lack of equity for families that had long carried the unreimbursed burden of care for their elderly but because family care was disappearing.

This has led to the prediction that nursing home placements may be utilized for an even greater percentage of the elderly in the future. Legislative proposals in 1983 focused on families being required to help fund nursing home placement rather than providing them funds to keep the elderly at home.

The reasons for decreased family care of the elderly are as follows:

- Families are smaller and there are fewer grown children to share the burden of caring for an aged parent.
- People live longer; the very old elderly (75 and up) are the most rapidly growing part of the population. Therefore, there are more dependent elderly to care for than ever before.
- The stable family, living geographically near the older generation members and in a home large enough to accommodate an extra person, no longer is the norm. Houses are smaller or have been replaced by apartments; the wife often is a full-time wage earner and unable to monitor an aged person during the day; families are more mobile and often far away from the elderly person's home ground.

Because of these demographic changes it is becoming more likely that elderly persons will be institutionalized as they become dependent and live increasingly longer. One researcher reports that the biggest reason for nursing home placement in New York City is patients' inability to walk (HSA, 1977).

Institutionalization's Costs Higher

Institutionalization nearly always is more expensive than home care in terms of public funds. The hidden costs of family care have not been part of that formula; room and board, clothing, and lost wages of family caretakers all are expenses lost in such a comparison. To avoid huge increases of public expenditures for care of the elderly, federal policy must consider subsidizing or substituting for family care, or pay less of the nursing home costs.

If home care is to be continued as a less costly alternative to institutionalization, then the availability of such services must be increased. Because of the restrictive nature of Medicare home health care eligibility, the availability and access to services have dropped slowly but consistently following an initial rise (Ricker-Smith & Trager, 1974; Somers, 1978). It has been estimated that a quarter to a third of all nursing home beds are filled with patients who could be cared for at home (Allen, 1974; Vladeck, 1980). However, those estimates are based on adequate supply of home health services and continued family assistance, none of which are likely to be available in the necessary amounts in the future without changes in public policy.

WELFARE AND HEALTH POLICY

As to the fourth finding, the nation's views of welfare and health policy must become less rigid and compartmentalized. This artificial division causes conflicts in Medicare aims for home care. Historically, public health and welfare benefits have been differentiated—those for health being medical care aimed at curing illness and those for welfare being the social services such as housing subsidies, food stamps, and homemakers.

Vladeck (1980) traces the development of nursing homes as an "indoor" welfare benefit and describes how that welfare care became medical care when nursing homes came under the aegis of hospitals in Hill-Burton legislation in 1954. Nursing homes, however, continue to be institutions for the frail and dependent elderly, who are not necessarily ill.

It is becoming clear that home care cannot substitute for institutional treatment without support services (Vladeck, 1980). Other writers have noted that most morbidity is of a chronic nature and that a combination of services is needed. Vicente Navarro (1974) writes:

The division of health services into two branches, curative and preventive, hinders rather than helps health workers who provide the care.

Today we have a structure where acute care is separated from chronic care, hospital care from ambulatory care, preventive medicine from curative medicine and social from medical care—separations and divisions that are due more to the power of the special interest groups and historical inertia than to the rational distribution of resources required to take care of our populations. These anachronistic divisions are felt most acutely where integration of services is most needed in the care of our populations, most of whom are chronically diseased.

A policy framework is needed that is different from the existing purely process-oriented one. Instead of looking merely at the components of care, more emphasis should be given to the original outcome desired: to substitute home care services for institutionalization. In addition, the perspective on health vs. social benefits needs to be reexamined, for not only is the division somewhat arbitrary but the entitlement to certain services tends to result in expensive services' going to those not in need and in duplication of care for persons who receive both health and social welfare benefits. Costing out family care, which is fast disappearing, can provide data important for future public policy for long-term care.

REFERENCES

Allen, D. Agencies' perceptions of factors affecting home care referrals. *Medical Care,* October 1974, *12,* 828-844.

Berkman, L., & Syme, L. Social networks, host resistance, and mortality. *American Journal of Epidemiology,* November 1979, *109,* 186-204.

Brickner, P. The homebound aged: A medically reachable group. *Annals of Internal Medicine,* 1975, *82,* 1-6.

Callahan, J. Responsibilities of families for their severely disabled elders. *Health Care Financing Review,* Winter 1980, *1*(3), 29-48.

Clinton, C. *Local success and federal failure.* Cambridge, Mass.: ABT Books, 1979.

Davis, K. *Lessons of Medicare and Medicaid for national health insurance.* Washington, D.C.: 1974.

Donabedian, A. *A guide to medical care administration.* New York: American Journal of Public Health Press, 1969, 3-5.

Feder, J. Medicare implementation and the policy process. *Journal of Health Policy, Politics & Law,* Summer 1977, 173-189.

Gary, L.R. *Home health care regulation: Issues and opportunities.* New York: Hunter College, 1979.

Hammond, J. Home health care cost effectiveness: An overview of the literature. *Public Health Reports,* July-August 1979, 305-311.

Home care in New York state. Albany, N.Y.: Home Care Association of New York State, May 1979.

Home health care: Its utilization, costs, and reimbursement. New York: Health Services Agency of New York City, November 1977.

Home health: The need for a national policy to better provide for the elderly. Department of Health, Education, and Welfare, Report to Congress, December 1977, p. 24.

Kingsdale, J. Marrying regulatory and competitive approaches to health care cost containment. *Journal of Health Policy, Politics & Law,* Spring 1978, *4*(1), 20-42.

Kurowski, B. *Cost per episode of home health care: Executive summary.* Boulder, Colo.: University of Colorado Center for Health Services Research (CHSR), March 1979.

Lavor, J., & Callender, M. Home health cost effectiveness: What are we measuring? *Medical Care,* October 1976, *14,* 866-872.

Navarro, V. From public health to health of the public. *American Journal of Public Health,* June 1974, *64,* 538-542.

Omaha VNA. *A classification system for client problems in community health nursing.* (Department of Health and Human Services, Public Health Service. Washington, D.C.: U.S. Government Printing Office, June 1980.

Pegels, C. *Health care and the elderly.* Rockville, Md.: Aspen Systems Corporation, 1980.

Ricker-Smith, K., & Trager, B. In-home health services in California. *Medical Care,* March 1978, 266.

Smith, B., & Hollander, N. (Eds.). *Medicare: A shared responsibility.* Washington, D.C.: National Academy of Public Administration, 1973.

Somers, A. The high cost of health care for the elderly: Diagnosis, prognosis, and some suggestions for therapy. *Journal of Health Policy, Politics & Law,* Summer 1978, *4*(2), 163-180.

VanDyke, F., & Elliott, R. *Military Medicare.* Washington, D.C.: U.S. Department of Defense, 1969.

VanDyke, F., & Brown, V. Organized home care. *Inquiry,* June 1972, 3-16.

Vladeck, B. *Unloving care.* New York: Basic Books, Inc., 1980.

Weissert, W. *Long-term care: Health in the U.S.* NCHSR, 1979.

Weissert, W. *Effects and costs of day care and homemaker services for the chronically ill elderly.* NCHSR, February 1980.

Chapter 8

Health Services and the Policy Process

Policy involves decisions to allocate resources for a given endeavor or outcome. Public policy is the allocation of public resources. Health policy in America has been broadly shaped by public allocation of resources.

There are two major areas of health policy in the United States: biomedical and health services. Biomedical policy is concerned with the use of medical technology, drugs, and procedures to limit the presence or sequellae of disease. The findings from biomedical research are reflected regularly in policy. For example, policy supports a treatment that research shows to be efficacious either through funding to encourage the use of that specific therapy or by making opportunities available for professionals to learn how to provide them.

Health services research, however, has not had such a clear impact on policy formation. Health services research is concerned with the relationship between consumers and providers of health care and how that care is influenced by organization, technology, financing, and payment. It essentially is social sciences research, dealing with the behavior of professionals and clients under varying systems of organization and financing. It has been federally funded only since 1963 and therefore is a much newer endeavor than biomedical research. The advent of Medicare strengthened the federal focus on health services research, particularly on the organization and distribution of care to the poor and the aged.

Research in health services tends to influence the climate in which decisions are made rather than to bring about specific changes in policy. It does so by highlighting ideas, trends, and issues and thereby making it more likely for policymakers to be aware of desirable options for change. Whenever the logical outcome is a shift of resources from one group to another, the impact of such research is lessened by the strong political focus of the status quo beneficiaries (Mechanic, 1974). "Logical" changes become operational quickly only when no one loses anything from the proposed change.

The importance of this relationship cannot be overstated in view of the direction of health services policy development in the early 1980s. Health services research has been used primarily to justify existing policies by describing or evaluating them. Developmental research has been less common and limited mainly to demonstration projects funded for the usual reason of cost containment alternatives (e.g., the nursing home without walls, nurse practitioners, physician extender projects, homemaker services for the elderly homebound). The trend continues for funding of "relevant" research (related to existing policy) in contrast to developmental (Gibson, 1978).

PROBLEMS IN LINKING RESEARCH AND POLICY

The research-policy relationship in health services is complex because the field is strongly multidisciplinary; is based on a data base that is highly imperfect, with few definitive answers; and it addresses a subject area in which there is more consensus on goals than on methodology.

The health field is dominated by physicians, both as the primary caregivers and as gatekeepers to the access to nearly all other services, including institutionalization, referrals to other professionals, and diagnostic studies. There are, however, other disciplines regularly involved in the delivery of services, including health facility administrators, physiotherapists and other rehabilitation professionals, nurses, social workers, medical suppliers, and pharmacists. Each group has a different perspective on care delivery, based on the values and services of its particular discipline.

The pharmaceutical industry, for example, focuses on providing safe and effective drugs while the nursing profession is more interested in safe, effective therapies that may be aimed more at self-care and life style changes than on drug therapy. Research findings from these two groups thus may be contradictory, not because of conflicting interpretation of facts but because different data are collected with different aims in mind.

Weakness in the Data Base

The data base in health services traditionally has been incomplete and imperfect. The mystique of the medical process has served to keep medical authority unchallenged and has promoted passivity and unquestioning compliance by patients. "The doctor knows best" may not be a false assumption but that attitude has inhibited the development of a data base from which the value of alternative treatments could be learned.

Similarly, quality in health care has not been well defined because it has been widely accepted that the professionals delivering the services were the ones who could best determine quality, so those being served did not need to be involved in that determination. Even as an objective data base on quality criteria and standards is developed, and cost-benefit and cost-effectiveness studies on health care delivery are carried out, the results will not provide definitive guidelines for policymakers. The answers to questions are not clear, with the result that decisions about treatment or the organization of care are based on individual values and preferences.

For instance, when biomedical research shows that in certain kinds of breast malignancy a lumpectomy is equally as life saving as a radical mastectomy, then the resulting policy for treatment protocols is developed with little dissent. Surgeons continue giving care, and the procedure changes, but the system and rewards are not upset in any major way; patients therefore clearly benefit from the recommended option.

However, when research shows that health maintenance organizations (HMOs) provide safe, effective care with lower costs, the ensuing policy does not necessarily promote HMO development. The lag in policy development stems from two factors: (1) the physician lobby, which exerts pressure to maintain existing fee-for-service patient relationships, and (2) the patients themselves, who prefer to maintain the optimum freedom of choice regarding all of their caregivers and health facilities.

Routes to Goals Vary

There is a strong consensus regarding the goals of health services—safe, effective, high-quality care at the lowest cost possible. How to achieve those goals, however, depends on values and preferences as well as facts. The quality issue, in particular, is most difficult to judge and to weigh against the issues of cost and safety. HMOs' development, for example, has been delayed most by physicians and patients who cite lack of choice and therefore regard them as a less than optimum system of care delivery. The lack of a consensus on methodology, and an imperfect data base in health care also plague other efforts toward consistent national policy development in education and defense, for instance.

All national policy development shares problems of conflicting constituencies, limited resources, and the well-known tendency for entrenchment of the status quo. Even deliberate policy decisions have unforeseen consequences in development in other areas. One of the clearest examples is the development of nursing home policy (Vladeck, 1980), wherein social welfare policy broadly influenced health service delivery. These factors help to explain why health services policy often is fragmented, inconsistent, incremental, and favorable to current beneficiaries. They also explain why policy so rarely is related to research.

Recommendations from health services research often suggest changes in the practice of professionals or in the structure of the organizations in which they work. These recommendations, although they may appear to be logical and beneficial, rarely become policy because changes in practice and organization of service delivery are complex, time consuming, and costly. Changes in professional practice may require new relationships or a shifting of responsibilities or the surrender of valued prerogatives or activities. Organizational reforms may appear clearly justified but, again, the complexity of change required makes reforms less likely.

The status quo factor is the natural tendency of professionals and administrators to continue what they have been doing. Change is always suspect, particularly when recommendations call for major shifts in resources and new ways of going about work. Since physicians, in particular, exert a major influence on health services policy development, their traditional relationships and mode of practice are so rewarding personally they have a great incentive against change.

The policy changes flowing from biomedical research have a different impact on professional practice. Usually such findings point to discrete incremental changes in the provision of services, such as new chemotherapy protocols or revised surgical procedures. These kinds of changes do not disrupt existing relationships and authority but rather tend to strengthen and enhance them.

Successful reforms are those that are acceptable to the individuals or groups most benefited by the existing system and that also are congruent with values in the society. Reforms aimed at increasing preventive self-care or at limiting access to high technology services have been received poorly at the policy-making level. Most constituents of policymakers value existing patterns of care even though research may show that they are ineffective or overly costly. The American society in particular values high technology and passive curative care.

THOSE WHO PAY THE PIPER CALL THE TUNE

René Dubos wrote, more than two decades ago, "To ward off disease or recover health, men as a rule find it easier to depend on the healers than to attempt the more difficult task of living wisely" (Dubos, 1959). The preference for the very best, most comprehensive, and technologically superior care predominates among individuals in society. As long as recipients of care choose and pay for their own services, and liberal insurance coverage disguises the costs to them, the pattern of increasingly sophisticated and expensive care will continue.

However, if payment shifts from the private to the public sector, the direction of health care policy will change. What individuals buy for themselves is not necessarily what they will buy for others. As more and more health care is paid for with public dollars, and as federal costs of existing programs continue to escalate, the use (and therefore the availability) of sophisticated and costly services may decline. Taxpayers question where their money goes, and by limiting what the public programs pay for, the development of those very services is limited for everyone. This may or may not be "good."

Limitation of dollar investment may deter broad availability of new or costly therapies but may allow for those diverted resources to be used in even more beneficial ways. For example, taxpayers can choose for themselves whether to have elective surgery such as a hip replacement or expensive diagnostic work such as a cardiac catheterization and will knowingly forgo a new car or home improvements to do so. However, if they are asked, through public policy allocation, to subsidize those same services for everyone, and in doing so implicitly agree to divert public funds from the development of car safety or inexpensive solar heating developments from which they could benefit personally, then it becomes less likely that those services will be made available.

Since the late 1970s, the trend has been toward decreasing the federal role in the delivery of health services. A major factor was the economy; there was less latitude for use of federal monies than before and the resources were less plentiful.

FEDERAL POLICY AND LOCAL OUTCOMES

There also is evidence of federal policy's being manipulated to serve local priorities. Clinton's study (1979) of a rural southern community development project shows that strict eligibility for federal funding could be met at the local level but still provide wide latitude for use of those monies, resulting in lack of correlation between federal intent and local application. Another example was the long-term patient (mentioned in Chapter 3) who was transferred 28 times between funding sources in the course of his care by one agency (DHEW, 1979).

Ginzberg (1977), writing on health reform, makes it clear that the answers for policy decisions will come from solutions developed locally—partly because the service needs of the future must be delivered in family settings (for reasons of economy and need) and partly because services are delivered locally, to individuals, and therefore local know-how and resources are necessary for solving local needs.

Vladeck (1977) writes of the problems inherent in health planning legislation that impose state and local costs without regard for local resources. Vladeck strengthens the argument for a stronger local role in policy development by stressing how future policy will be influenced strongly by existing autonomous functions at the state level (insurance regulation and health care facility regulation) and by the impact of the structure of federalism (sharing of powers among the three levels of government).

Traditionally it has been thought that national policy leads to a predictable local outcome. Clinton (1979) makes it clear that this "impact" theory needs reexamination in light of his findings in his rural development study. That analysis documents the deliberate use of federal monies for very different local outcomes than was the intent of the funding. He concludes that the same unpredictable outcomes can occur even when the manipulation is less deliberate. Vladeck's nursing home policy studies agree with this analysis.

Nursing home policy never has been developed directly but always has been an offshoot of welfare and health approaches. Many of the problems in nursing home care arise from the deficits in meeting needs of their patients and in failure to address that industry for what it has become—a huge provider of care for the elderly population, with the great majority of providers being in the private (for-profit) sector yet relying on public funds for much of their income.

The route from federal policy to local implementation may not be as clear or predictable as had been thought. Local decision making influences the efficiency and effectiveness of national health policy. If the outcomes of policy are to be reliable and valid, the actual implementation process at the service delivery level must be known and measured. Local "manipulation" must be known if the outcomes measured are related to the actual processes carried out. This relationship in turn can be used in policy analysis and policy changes.

There are indications that this may be happening already. The underdevelopment of home health agencies has been attributed in part to the absence of start-up funds; of stable, continuing funding; and of fiscal policies to cover inflationary cost increases, staff "down time," and unpredictable reimbursement (Trager, 1971).

Although many of the Health Care Financing Administration (HCFA) cost control policies on Medicare reimbursement for home health services seem to be arbitrary and based on cost containment alone (e.g., cost caps without regard to demographic differences, travel barriers, or alternative resources), the agency has taken steps to become responsive to some of these variables. For instance, the HCFA schedule on limits of home health agency costs per visit has adjustments built in for inflation, regional wage rates, and urban vs. nonurban agencies. These regulations have broad implications for agency and service growth. This acknowledgment of the importance of local factors is encouraging for further policy development.

CONTINUED NEED FOR FEDERAL POLICY

Although the trend in health services delivery was toward a reduced federal role, the changes were more likely in the administration and evaluation of care than in the funding. Initial Reagan administration efforts to decentralize government, including requiring the states to assume many health and welfare benefit programs, ran into difficulties, including problems involving the release of funds to the states and their divergence (primarily) to the military. States were loathe to increase taxes to maintain services under such a transfer of authority. As funding became ever tighter and providers were pressed to deliver increasingly more goods and services, there would be hard choices to be made.

One of the biggest issues was the cost of health care:

1. It is very expensive, with costs rising out of proportion to the ability to fund them.
2. Those who need the most care—the aged and the poor—are least able to pay for it themselves.
3. The aged as a percentage of the population are growing.

The federal government, having assumed the major responsibility for the health care of the poor and the aged through Medicare and Medicaid, found that those programs were consuming far more than anticipated. Rather than face the tough ethical issues involved in cutbacks, or the tough political issues in changing the delivery system, the course of action chosen was to hand those problems and responsibilities over to the states but with only a fraction of the needed resources.

At state and local levels issues become more politicized and single issues can become disproportionately persuasive. Short-term interests may be more likely to win out and the needs of the disenfranchised or the powerless are less likely to be met. These inequities occur because local governments serve local needs, and influences can be closer and more personal, and thus potentially more effective when legislative priorities are set and fund allocations are made. The needs of the aged and the poor, in particular, tend to be low priority at that level because those groups have a weak power base and traditionally are less involved. Only when the economic climate is favorable, and times are good enough for a variety of programs, will the needs of the less powerful be met.

At the federal level, legislators can develop a broader perspective on needs and can be somewhat more removed from local pressures—but they still have to go home to the voters to be reelected and those voters can have their own ideas on national needs and priorities that can affect what their senators and representatives do in Congress.

The broader aim of Congress is to provide for the well-being of the nation as a whole. Programs that might not develop in any local area nonetheless can be needed in most of the nation. If isolated states subsidized health care, that would have been an incentive for the aged in other states to move where their service needs would be covered by government (state, in this case). As more and more of the elderly swelled the populations where such coverage existed, those states quickly would lose the ability to provide those services. Therefore, not only would inequities occur but the programs themselves would be doomed.

Some services are possible only if everyone contributes equally with the assurance that no funding group (the taxpayers) will be overburdened. This is true of Medicare and Medicaid, and the latter leaves part of the decision on coverage to the local areas that cofund the services. Both Medicare and Medicaid were preceded by isolated state programs that funded health care for the aged and the poor. However, those programs were spotty and often functioned in the areas of greatest resources and least need. Where there are high percentages of the elderly and the poor (or of children, another traditionally disadvantaged group), there usually is a low tax base as well. Therefore, where need is highest, resources are lowest, and the inequities increase.

No one group wants the responsibility (or has the ability) for providing services from which everyone benefits, such as clean air or national defense. There thus must be a consensus and common participation if certain services or programs are to become available.

The federal government, as noted, not only provides a vantage point for developing a broader perspective on needs and equity it also has broader interests as priorities. If care is provided inequitably, the result is lower average health status for the nation. Inequities of any kind tend to provoke hostility, bitterness, and, potentially, violence. The preservation of peace and well-being clearly are in the nation's best interests.

For all these reasons the federal government will continue to serve as a social conscience for its citizens and, it is to be hoped, will assure the most equitable provision of the nation's resources. Acknowledgment that individual states cannot serve that larger purpose suggests that programs that serve the needs of large populations who are nowhere top priority for action should be maintained at the federal level.

Federalism (the sharing of powers among federal, state, and local governments) traditionally supported state sovereignty. In the last few decades in the United States there was a steady growth of federal assumption of programs. With the Reagan administration's "new federalism" approach of turning numerous programs over to the states, there was a need for health professionals in particular to publicize the somewhat different perspective essential if services were to be provided to disadvantaged populations. Programs needed by a great number of people, but which lack local support should remain at the federal level, at least for funding and for the assurance of availability and access for every eligible person.

PROCESS AND OUTCOME STRATEGIES

The arguments for the "new federalism" were that services should be developed locally in order to meet local needs and to use local resources most effectively. It also was designed to make possible closer evaluation by those who provided the funds—the states.

These arguments were very persuasive because:

- The impact theory of policy was coming under question.
- Manipulation of policy was more likely when the buyer and evaluator of services was distant and essentially anonymous.
- Needs and resources did differ substantially in different regions in the country.

Perhaps a more legitimate emphasis on sharing rather than shifting power would better fit the public's needs, at least in the area of health services. The federal government could establish the broad aims of programs, develop methods of assuring availability and access to the target population, and use tax funds to pay for them. State or local governments would develop the process of giving care best suited to the resources and needs of particular locales. Evaluation of such programs would focus on whether their broad aims were met, whether those entitled to care received it, whether funds were used efficiently, and whether quality and patient satisfaction were promoted. This would leave a good deal of flexibility at the local level concerning how to use funds to promote the program objectives.

This proposal is a choice between current health policy, which provides that a certain process should be followed, and a different kind of policy that stresses that a certain outcome should be achieved. Not only is the latter less able to be manipulated, it also allows for and requires the kind of creative freedom that professionals engage in, regardless of policy.

Outcome-oriented programs are less likely to be manipulated for a number of reasons:

- Professionals adjust health policy so they can give the care needed. If there were no policy dictating the elements of professional practice there would be far less reason to tinker with criteria.
- Progress toward an outcome (such as health status) can be assessed at given times during the process by an independent evaluator, again keeping manipulation at a minimum. Evaluation of process criteria is much more difficult and open to'interpretation. For example, how can an evaluator judge the validity of homebound status or need for skilled care on one visit, especially if the caregiver chooses to obscure the evidence?
- Professionals using outcome goals are working toward a condition that clearly is beneficial to the patient—the prevention of orthopedic deformities or the maintenance of independence in daily living activities. These goals are more universally valued by the professionals giving the care, and therefore less likely to be manipulated. Process criteria, on the other hand, have fewer elements that are directly related to patient well-being or that can be evaluated

easily; therefore, they are more likely to be adapted to meet the professional commitment to the care given.

The overall aims, broad-based funding capacity, and objective evaluations of effectiveness and quality are federal functions. They assure accountability to the public payers and good, equitable service to consumers (the public). There still is wide latitude for professionals to provide services they may decide on individually and for communities or states to determine priorities of care availability. For instance, federally financed health care in North Dakota might include patients' transportation expenses whereas in New York City the same program might cover nutrition assistance instead. The difference in need (family availability or distance to health care facilities) would dictate different service coverage.

This proposed change in health policy can promote cost containment. If the policy of funding given services were to continue, costs could only rise. The unit price of a given service is not likely to decrease, a factor that is even more true where high technology and ultraskilled expensive caregivers are the norm. The number of high-use health care consumers also is growing fast. Initial cost containment could be achieved within existing policy by restricting eligibility, but there was a distinct possibility that these individuals' health needs would not disappear just because their insurance did. This would produce no saving of public money; it would only be a switch from one program to another: from health coverage to welfare coverage.

With outcome-oriented policy, a great deal of creativity is possible for finding more efficient ways of keeping people healthy and independent. Instead of eligibility's being locked into certain given services, it could be determined by the potential for reaching certain outcomes. Under existing policy, for instance, patients may receive expensive professional care for weeks, not because those services are helping them achieve independence but because they are the legitimate access to other needed care. Under an outcome system, reimbursable care would be determined by what was needed to achieve the desired health status. In some cases it might be professional services, in others only homemaker or nurse's aide help might be required.

INCREASED HOME CARE CAN SAVE COSTS

Medicare home health services are of particular importance in the research and policy area in the immediate future because of the growing concern for cost containment.

Hospital expenses rose even faster than other health care costs since Medicare's beginning. Technological sophistication was only a part of the reason. Professional salaries also rose quickly for both independent practitioners and those salaried by hospitals. Insurance premiums were up, and higher costs for institutions' maintenance functions such as fuel oil and electricity contributed to the problem. Clearly institutional care, and hospitals in particular, were in line for continued cost containment policy. If home care services that will prevent hospitalization could be developed (and reimbursed), Medicare will have achieved a major cost saving.

INCREMENTALISM LIMITS CHANGE

An incremental approach is one where many small but related steps are taken serially to advance. Because policy tends to be incremental and protective of the current system and beneficiaries, its development tends not to take new directions, even when incrementalism is not working. Often the new directions are not followed because the political power of those defending the status quo overrides ''logical'' reforms.

For example, the increase in acute care technology has dramatically changed mortality figures for common serious pathology. Detection, drug therapy, and sophisticated monitoring and resuscitation have reduced the mortality from acute myocardial infarction sharply. Cardiac bypass and transplant surgery have further decreased morbidity and premature death. Life support systems have compensated for acute damage until patients have recovered sufficiently to live independently again.

Increased and expanded resort to these technologies quite naturally has led to their use for prolonging life that is not capable of being restored, so instead of a positive achievement, patients often experience extended and costly morbidity even though death has been delayed. The argument can be made that life of low quality is preferable to no life, but the issue is not that simple. Life at low quality—a blind, diabetic 80-year-old man on kidney dialysis, for example—cannot be seen in isolation. Policy that provides for that kidney dialysis allocates resources that could be committed elsewhere—toward readers for blind students, or highway safety, or research on improving the quality of life for the elderly. Trade-offs are inherent in every policy decision and choices rarely are simple or straightforward. The incremental approach which works so smoothly in policy development, however, is chiefly responsible for the overuse of existing therapies or organizational process.

By building on what already exists more efficient and useful modalities sometimes are bypassed. For example, using the SSA claims processing system for payment of Medicare bills was probably costly and inadequate for value judgments such as quality. Awareness of this flaw in current policy development can avoid some of the problems in such a process. Instead of building vertically on policy rooted in another time with other priorities, horizontal thinking is required.

Are the needs the same? Have values changed? Are there different resources now? Answering these questions will not, alone, provide workable direction for policy development but will produce information needed for the ultimate decisions.

DEVELOPMENT OF NEW POLICY

Once the current needs, priorities, and resources are identified, they must be developed into policy that continues to benefit recipients of the existing system. For instance, cost-containment policy in hospitals has met with success where the facilities have some control over maintaining their profits; prospective reimbursement per hospitalization episode is more acceptable than ceilings imposed on per diem repayment. Where hospitals receive a given dollar amount for the care of a patient admitted for a specific medical condition, there is some freedom in how they spend that money on care, producing a great incentive for efficiency. Where per diem reimbursement is cut, hospitals are more likely to extend the service delivery time to make up for revenues lost during the acute care phase—an incentive for inefficiency. There also must be incentives for physicians if they are to alleviate the inadequate rural and inner city availability of medical care.

Successful policy development therefore depends on acknowledging the political necessity of providing rewards to current beneficiaries and on using the horizontal thinking required to assure that the incremental approach is building services that are needed and valued and for which the necessary resources are available. If these two guidelines are followed, it is more likely that new policy directions can be successful. The public is much more likely to accept different allocations of resources when new needs are demonstrated and when its own benefits are protected.

The Perils of Short-Term Action

Another policy step that must be avoided is the seductive appeal of opting for an action or solution that is not desired for the long term but seems to be the only possible step forward at the time. This kind of short-term "it's better than nothing" action is dangerous. When Medicare was initiated the Social Security Administration was designated as the claims processor since it had a system in place for those same beneficiaries, even though health services constituted a kind of benefit very different from cash assistance. Rather than delaying Medicare implementation to allow for the development of a claims processing operation that would look at appropriateness and quality of service, the quick and easy way was adopted. This action was responsible in part for the deficits in assessing quality and appropriateness of care that allowed fraud and abuse to develop. Quality and appropriateness of service also suffered because of the decision not to address the process of medical care. This was omitted in order to gain physician support for the legislation.

The Nursing Home Bed Issue

These beginning positions very quickly became entrenched and continued to be difficult to change. Any policy decision becomes solidified and buttressed by its very presence and the interests of those involved. Such short-sighted policy was under consideration for nursing home beds and for nurse practitioner licensure.

By early 1980, the number of nursing home beds had been nearly the same for some time; few new beds were developed because different alternatives were being sought for care of the debilitated elderly. During the search for new options the number of elderly needing that kind of care burgeoned, and the pressures for providing services to them were great.

One alternative to nursing home placement is the Nursing Home without Walls, or the Long-Term Home Health Care Program (LTHHCP) signed into law in New York State as Chapter 895 (1977). It establishes Medicaid payment for nursing home eligible Medicaid beneficiaries to receive that care at home instead. Savings accrue to federal and state coffers because services for LTHHCP cannot exceed 75 percent of what traditional nursing home costs would be per month. The easy answer would be build more nursing home beds until another alternative could be developed. However, once that alleviated the demand for care, the pressure to develop alternatives would have been weakened and the status quo strengthened even though it might not be the ultimate service desired (Vladeck, 1980).

Nursing Licensure

A similar situation existed with nurse practitioner licensure. Expanded nursing practice (physical examinations and treatment of uncomplicated illness) may or may not be covered under existing nurse licensure laws. As of 1983 a number of states, including New York, have proposals for separate Nurse Practitioner licensure. Legal opinions vary over the need, and caution predominates in the courts and in new legislation. There is no accepted line at which nurses legitimately treating health problems for which their license covers them step over into the realm of medicine. That line will probably eventually be drawn over diagnosis of pathology and some prescriptive therapies (some drugs, and some lab and x-ray work). Even where there is overlap between nurse practitioner/physician practice, such as diet counseling for hypertension, or treatment of an upper respiratory infection or well-child guidance, the positive aspects of nurse practitioner practice (increased access for underprivileged populations and lower costs, for instance) make it less likely that nurses will be legislated out of participation in such service delivery.

Licensure proposals were developed that are acceptable to physicians and legislators, but at a price for nurses—they would place expanded nursing practice under the authority of physicians. Although this would protect nurse practitioners from possible charges of practicing outside their licensure restrictions, it would move nursing from an autonomous professional status to that of medical assistance, which nurses obviously would regard as a negative step for their profession and for society.

Policy decisions tend to become lasting even though their intent often is contrary to the resulting law. If nursing were to accept physician direction for expanded practice, the profession could change substantially. Ironically, the intent of expanding nursing would serve instead to establish a law that would decrease professional status.

Accountability and Alternatives

Policymaking is always imperfect in assuring that the best use of resources for the most desired outcome is achieved. The total trade-offs in resources and in goals cannot be known, yet accountable policymaking demands a thoughtful assessment of alternate uses of resources and potential alternate outcomes. This accountability is particularly important in the public sector, where resources emanate from many who are not beneficiaries—Medicare, for instance, is funded for the elderly and the disabled through a tax on every worker's salary.

When the buyer of a service is the recipient of it, which is characteristic of private sector relationships, policy can be developed so that only the seller and buyer are satisfied. A greater responsibility is required in providing goods and services purchased with public money. Even with the full acceptance of such responsibility, the system is complex since these publicly funded services usually are not provided by public agencies, at least not in the United States where the private sector delivers the great majority of services.

Instead, private sector providers contract to deliver services and that sector tends to favor providers, not recipients. Government acknowledges the accountability inherent in the use of public dollars, but if the care is not delivered through a public agency, supervision and evaluation to protect that trust are difficult. Two traditional methods are employed to assure compliance with federal authority. One is ownership, the public utility model, in which the public owns the service provider and has a direct method of assuring accountability. This is not prevalent in the United States. The other is regulation of the rates of private providers.

INSURANCE—A MAJOR COST FACTOR

In addition to these complexities, health services recipients traditionally have been accepting of what providers say they need. To further weaken the incentives for recipients to evaluate services the majority of care is covered by insurance and therefore is a cost hidden to them. Insurance coverage effectively reduces the price barrier for use; if one premium covers the services, then consumers look only at that figure and, as noted, in most cases even it is a hidden cost, usually paid as an employee benefit. Insurance rates, although regulated by the states, usually can be approved at higher rates if it can be shown that costs are up and increased premiums would be required to cover costs. Conversely, when insurance coverage costs go down, there is evidence that even then the carriers tend not to reduce premiums but instead broaden coverage to justify the old, high premium.

For example, when Medicare was enacted almost the entire population over age 65 came under the federal blanket, removing them for the most part from Blue Cross coverage. Since Blue Cross, like most insurance companies, is experience rated, the cost of insuring its remaining beneficiaries (still in the millions) dropped. Experience-rated coverage means that an individual premium within the population insured by the company is based on the average claims of that group: if an average policyholder claims $1,200 in benefits in one year, then each policyholder in that group will pay a premium of $1,200 plus a percentage of the company's administrative costs and other overhead. Since the elderly are disproportionately high users of health services, Blue Cross premiums should have dropped when those individuals were removed from its rolls. However, the rates did not drop—they stayed the same and coverage for remaining beneficiaries was broadened to cover expanded services.

Incentives for Constraint Lacking

Policy incentives for cost containment are lacking in the insurance industry and in consumer groups, both because of the coverage system and because users' behavior regarding health care differs from that involving the purchase of other goods and services. Patients do not examine health care recommendations very thoroughly, and it is providers, not consumers, who determine use of services— prescription of drugs and treatments, admission to hospitals, surgery, and the schedule of return visits.

Since consumers accept their incomplete knowledge and lack of independence in initiating and evaluating their health care, providers wield a disproportionate influence in service delivery. It has long been felt that the responsibility for quality in health care lies with the professionals who provide it. Quality cannot be legislated because, in most instances, the health care professionals are the only ones with sufficient knowledge to understand the comparative value of different treatments. This mystique has resulted in physicians' serving in an unparalleled position in policy structure: they determine what services will be provided, who will receive them, how often they can receive them, and whether the care is sufficient and of high quality.

Confronting a Dichotomy

Only since the government has become a major payer of health care bills (since Medicare and Medicaid were enacted) has there been any concerted public effort to influence health policy. Furthermore, since a large percentage of the nation's costs of care now is paid for with federal dollars, health policy increasingly will be developed to meet the standards of overall public policy, including assessment of appropriateness, cost effectiveness, and careful comparisons of alternate use of resources or alternate goals. These factors were not considered in the traditional delivery of health services; the overriding principle was to provide the optimum available care in every instance. Health professionals in particular have a commitment to give the best, most comprehensive care possible to every person who needs it. This results in an inherent dichotomy, with the government payer focusing on cost effectiveness and alternative uses of resources and with health professionals most concerned with furthering scientific knowledge of preventive, curative, and health maintenance care and the assured provision of those services to all possible beneficiaries.

Because public money is paying for more and more health care, public policy must be developed to resolve many of these conflicts. Not only should there be a compromise between public and professional interests but decisions must be made in the larger arena of publicly funded services. The most important decisions involve where health policy fits within other national priorities. Health care in the 1982 fiscal year claimed 10.4 percent of the GNP. Some analysts predicted it would account for 12 percent of GNP by the turn of the century (Pegels, 1980).

WHAT SERVICES TO INCLUDE?

To decide on health expenditures in the national budget, there first must be some consensus as to what services to include. Are they only those delivered or supervised by health professionals, or are they any services that enhance health? The latter category could include food, better housing, and homemaker services. Clearly a health budget that included those items would be far greater than one that covered only traditional care by providers. This may appear to be an unlikely issue to argue yet it has been around since 1965 because Medicaid services often are very different from the traditional approach under Medicare. Whereas Medicare services must be related to an acute medical condition and be ordered by a physician, Medicaid in some states covers purely custodial and comfort measures, e.g., home attendants in New York City, or homemakers in other areas.

Health services, unlike educational and defense components of the federal budget, are difficult to compartmentalize. Do they include preventive and maintenance services? Homemakers, meals on wheels, and transportation to a health facility in some instances can preserve health or prevent illness. Considering the costs of curative care, those other services might be a wise investment for federal dollars. However, if care were to include those measures as well as curative treatment, the money spent on health services would rise even faster.

Health policy determines not only what health care includes but how it is to be paid for. The fee-for-service system is clearly inflationary and has all the deficiencies of a process-oriented approach. Two key proposals of the Reagan administration's efforts to reduce federal health care costs were to place limits on reimbursement through prospective rates, and to increase cost sharing by patients covered by federal insurance.

The first approach is prospective reimbursement to institutions for care based on the patient's medical diagnosis and functional status. This system, called diagnosis-related groupings (DRGs), allows hospitals to use the predetermined payment in the most effective way to provide needed care. Prospective reimbursement offers incentives for provider efficiency but an unresolved question was whether it included adequate safeguards for patients so they would not be denied needed care. The government adopted prospective reimbursement as the method of paying for hospitalization of Medicare patients in 1982. In 1983, regulations were being developed which would acknowledge cost differences in teaching hospitals, small vs. large hospitals and urban vs. rural hospitals.

The second cost containment effort focused on patient copayment to reduce utilization rather than on provider incentives for efficiency. Under this plan, called the "competitive" approach to reducing health care costs (Davis, 1981), copayments and deductibles would be increased so that a lesser cost burden would fall on the insurer (such as the federal government, under Medicare). With consumers paying greater out-of-pocket costs, federal costs could be decreased and a decrease in utilization of services could be expected.

That system, too, presented problems. If patients denied themselves needed care because their own part of the cost was prohibitive, their unmet needs could result in an increase in expensive illness and rehabilitative care. And those costs (which usually are greater than the originally needed but neglected care) ultimately would be paid from the public purse for those who had no money. Not only would there be no ultimate public saving, there could well be a net loss. In addition, the competitive approach has long been recognized as being inequitable since it usually requires the same dollar amount payment from rich or poor consumers; no graduated-by-income deductible has been introduced.

Patients' Self-Promotion of Health

The third and complex approach would provide care not only according to need but also according to individual patients' participation in their health promotion;

e.g., surgical and chemotherapy and radiation therapy are effective in the cure or delayed mortality from lung cancer but they also are very expensive.

Some would suggest that federal dollars be spent for this care only when the patients did not smoke—those who smoked assumed the consequences of their known risk. This is not an easy solution. What of the mine workers who know the risks of lung disease but have no other option to make a living?

The idea of promoting better self-care (and, serendipitously, of lowering health care costs) is initially very attractive. However, blaming the victim can become an easy way for providers or insurers to shrug off their responsibilities in providing necessary care.

Productivity and Rehabilitation

A fourth approach to cost containment would be to limit federally funded care to services that will increase productivity, not only life saving but clearly rehabilitative. The rationale for this approach is that public dollars should be expended only for activities that will benefit the public, and those benefits should be demonstrable. Under such a limited economic perspective, a retired person who needs kidney dialysis or coronary bypass surgery would be denied those publicly funded services because the person no longer provided service to the community and as a retiree was a taker and not a contributor. Purely economic terms could reduce the human condition to such criteria. Even if the productivity concept were accepted, contribution to the community in any civilized nation must include more than economic measurement.

The wealth and value of experienced and aged nonworking citizens are hard to measure but easy to recognize. This group offers society not only the transmission of cultural values and access to experiential acumen but also a more tempered perspective on the nation's priorities. The economic productivity focus is important in this discussion of future Medicare policy, particularly in home health services, because the prolongation of life and healthful well-being of these citizens could well be determined solely on the basis of their contributions to the work force.

DIFFICULTIES IN A RATIONAL APPROACH

As has been noted, the policy process for health services is highly politicized. Because government is the payer for so many beneficiaries, policy development reflects specific political interests that stand to gain or lose by any reallocation of resources or change in funding priorities. These political factors tend to outweigh "logical" assessment of needs when policy is formulated. Professionals in particular may have difficulty accepting the primacy of political interests when their own knowledge and perspective clearly show that policy is taking the wrong direction—wrong in that it does not meet needs in the most efficient and useful way or wrong in that it does not meet priority needs at all.

Vladeck (1977, 1980) has identified two rules about policy that hamper a rational approach to planning: (1) there is no law that says policy must be consistent and (2) policy, once implemented, quickly tends to become entrenched, assuring that benefits will continue for both providers and beneficiaries. A third rule might be that policy more often favors political constituencies rather than demonstrated need.

If professionals are aware of these considerations they are more likely to be able to influence policy development. Because of their training and perspective, most professionals can determine health needs better than the legislators making policy. However, differing values about health care as well as vested interests in promoting their own disciplines lead to interprofessional lobbying. The group most likely to lose in such a test of influence is nursing. The reasons are many:

- Nursing traditionally has not had a solid, autonomous base. Being seen mainly as an arm of medicine has limited its voice in health policy development.
- The medical profession is less likely than ever to share its services to the public with nursing. The oversupply of physicians will serve to restrict the growth and spread of nursing professionalism. As physicians saturate the traditional curative and specialist field they are using their historical leadership position in medicine to move to include nursing's roles.
- Nursing's contributions to health status have always been difficult to measure. Most independent nursing activities are aimed at illness prevention, health promotion, and health maintenance. The outcomes of such activities rarely are visibly different from the health status that preceded the nursing intervention. Except in the area of health promotion, there may be no difference in health status. It is very difficult to measure or to value the absence of something—even when the thing avoided is very severe, such as stroke or cancer. One reason for this is that a tragedy avoided might never have happened anyway.

Because nursing so often provides these less dramatic services, the profession has less political clout in influencing policy or obtaining priority funding for that work, particularly to an extent commensurate with its value to society. Nursing should develop a political strategy to achieve acknowledgment of its leadership in directing its own activities and to win policy support for those services.

AN AGENDA FOR ACTION

An agenda for influencing policy development and implementation is essential:

1. The specific need to be met by policy must be defined clearly.
2. An assessment should be made as to whether the aim of policy not only fills a health need but also is valued by society.
3. A determination must be made whether additions to current policy will meet the need, or whether new directions are required.
4. Beneficiaries of existing policy must be identified if new direction is needed, as well as what they stand to lose if changes are made.
5. Some accommodations for lost benefits should be built into the new policy.
6. Short-term and long-term goals for policy outcomes must be determined.
7. Quality and appropriateness guarantees, necessary for public accountability, should be developed.
8. Incentives for cost containment must be provided.

Although this would seem to be a logical sequence for legislators to adopt, political interests can intervene at any step in the process. It is interesting to follow a specific issue through this maze. Nursing practice has expanded, in the nurse practitioner movement, to include health history taking, physical examinations to determine the presence of pathology, and management of uncomplicated illnesses. Although nurses have been doing this for more than 15 years, legislation to cover the practice explicitly has not evolved.

Many people believe that existing state nurse practice acts cover all nursing care that has been taught and that meets the legal criteria. Others believe that new activities should be covered explicitly, thereby requiring new licensure. Because some of the new nursing activities also are practiced by physicians, there is an argument over whether nurses should perform those functions under the supervision of doctors. Still others believe that new skills are regularly included under individual independent licensure and that simply because another practitioner also uses them does not confer supervisory status on the original user. For example, health educators are not required to practice under nursing supervision and nurses taking blood pressures need not practice under the supervision of physicians.

This issue has policy significance, for whoever has the autonomy to provide health histories, examinations, and illness management also will have the access, funding, and reimbursement for the delivery of those services. Policy will determine the benefits for providers and thus the availability of the services to consumers.

The need for the services is viewed differently by physicians, nurses, and the public. Physicians see the services as primarily medical and therefore to be provided only by doctors or under their auspices. Their view would preserve the existing illness orientation and high fee structure. Nurses, not uncharacteristically, do not agree, even among themselves, on the need for these skills. Some regard them as medical in purpose (illness detection and resolution) but as having now become part of independent nursing functions. Others see them as a way to provide nursing service, distinct from medical care. They identify the need to sanction expanded skills for nursing care—primarily health promotion, identification of illness risks with attendant preventive care, and the development and strengthening of healthful behaviors to maintain wellness. This group contends that the identification and management of uncomplicated illness is a secondary nursing goal.

Nurses therefore differ on the purpose of legislation for expanded skills, with one group wanting access to provide medical services and the others to expand existing nursing practice. The public most often views this new nursing practice as a duplication of the simpler aspects of medical practice. The public is familiar with and values illness resolution care and therefore accepts the safe and less expensive option of having competent nurses provide that service. The other clearly nursing services that can flow from the skills required in giving the familiar physical examinations are not well understood by the public and therefore not widely valued or sought. The primary desire of the public is to have a known service delivered safely at the least possible cost. To achieve that, the public generally is willing to accept and utilize nurses for that care.

Importance of Society's Interests

Policy direction already is confused at the first two steps in the preceding list— the needs definition and the consensus between policymakers and society. Political pressures can be decisive in such a conflict. Nursing, in order to be influential, will be more successful if it speaks to society's interests on this issue and does not simply espouse its own profession's desires.

For example, let it be assumed that nursing agreed (and that has to be the first step: agreement) that policy should sanction nurses' independently using examination and diagnostic skills to detect illness and that they could deliver those services less expensively than physicians. This focus would be acceptable to the public and therefore would detract from the power of organized medicine to have physicians supervise and bill for the nursing services.

If, on the other hand, nursing chose to focus on its traditional functions (teaching, prevention, promotion) that the new skills would enhance, the public would not be as strongly supportive of that view. Indeed, it might be swayed into thinking that nurses should be under physician direction if they used those skills in illness detection and management. If nursing could reach a consensus that the skills would be used for the consumer-valued services of illness care, there would be more chance that policy would be developed favoring nurse autonomy.

Cost and Access

Once it has been shown that nursing can carry out the services safely and appropriately, the other important issues for the public are cost and access. Nurses can provide the services for lower cost because they are not assuming the responsibility for acute care management or complex differential diagnosis, which physicians must shoulder even when performing on a less complicated level. As for access, nurses most likely will be providing these services in underserved medical areas anyway. Distribution of these services in such areas is more likely to increase if nurses perform them because the demand for lower cost care is not as great in areas of dense physician availability (which usually are wealthier).

By agreeing to offer service at lower cost and receiving greater access (along with providing illness resolution), nursing would have defined need in terms most likely for successful policy development. The next step would be to see whether new policy would be incremental, based on past policy, or whether new directions were needed.

Sanctioning these previously physician-only activities for nurses could be achieved easily by reinterpretation of existing state nurse practice acts or by amending the acts to cover such activities. The real problem, however, would be the threat to physician autonomy in illness care, and that could not be resolved easily. There would be a need to make sure the policy action somehow benefited physicians. A distinction must be made whereby physicians would maintain their autonomy for areas in which nurses did not have appropriate skills or judgment. In addition, there might be financial incentives built into reimbursement for collaborative practice between physicians and nurses. These moves cover items four and five in the agenda—recognition and recompense for lost benefits.

Short-Term and Long-Term Solutions

The easy short-term policy goal in the example analyzed here would be to have a law passed sanctioning the assumption of the new activities by nurses but placing them under physicians' supervision. Everyone would benefit: nurses could practice in the expanded role without fear of lawsuits and with assurance of payment; consumers would have more providers and potentially better access to these services; and physicians would maintain their traditional primacy.

In the long term, however, such a result would be counterproductive. Nursing would be in the position of reverting to subprofessional status; the fee for the "same" service surely would rise to meet the physician's level, especially if supervised by that doctor; access would not increase much because nurses could offer the services only where physician-supervisors already practiced; and the content of the care rarely would expand to include nursing measures. In this issue, as in many others, the easy approach could well be detrimental.

Quality, appropriateness, and cost containment would increasingly be necessary components of policy development. Quality and appropriateness measurements in this example also would serve to assure physicians and consumers that there would be safe and acceptable limits to the expansion of nursing practice. Cost containment can be one of the selling points for policy approving these new nursing skills.

The eight-point agenda in this example demonstrates that the policy decisions are political and arguable at every step. The process is a constant give-and-take among the public, the providers, and the representatives of both who make policy. The strategy steps are not nearly as important to learn as are the ways to influence that process, and this knowledge is key for professionals who want to affect the future of their practice.

Keys to Exerting Influence

Professionals influence policy best if they can speak to what is good for the consumers, especially in the areas of cost, quality, and access, and in describing the outcomes under different policy options. They can be successful in influencing policymaking by recognizing and using the political issues and by defusing any and all risks to established beneficiaries.

Hard data always are more dramatic and persuasive than value statements; for instance, it would be effective to publicize the fact that a health history and physical exam by a nurse practitioner costs, on average, only a third as much as the same service from a physician. Nurses again, in particular, can benefit from an objective and politically sophisticated approach to influencing policy decisions, knowing what both the hidden and the publicized issues are and knowing how to marshal facts that address both overt and covert arguments.

Similarly, it is vital to know whom to address with these arguments. Legislators are one bloc and consumer groups most affected by a specific policy action are another. Professionals must work to attain consensus among themselves, weighing the trade-offs that may be necessary to produce a successful, unified effort. Those who could be affected adversely by new policy also must be included in the discussion and lobbying efforts, and benefits for those who stand to lose should be considered.

This outlook and this strategy in policy development for home health services constitute a critical professional effort, especially for nurses. The recommendations that follow are based on this political and professional perspective. They also attempt to solve some of the important health needs of the aged.

Nursing to the Fore in Home Care

These recommendations suggest a policy that would place nurses rather than physicians in the position of directing home care services. The eight-point agenda outlined earlier made it clear that this policy proposal would be difficult to implement. The need for nurse-directed care is not widely recognized. Medically directed care is the only reimbursable health service available. However, the public was coming to recognize crisis-oriented care could be a lot more expensive than preventive services. This is especially true for the elderly, who often become completely disabled following an acute illness or trauma and who then may require full-time services. However, preventive or health maintenance care is reimbursable only in social-medical programs such as Medicaid or in some instances under HMO coverage.

Nurses provide these services in the course of medically directed home care, but there are few data showing the cost of preventive service without concurrent medical care. Some research shows that social networks and maintenance care decrease mortality and increase independence of the elderly (Berkman & Syme, 1979; Weissert, 1980) but the associated costs of such coverage have been projected as an add-on to the existing medical care system rather than projecting the cost of providing maintenance care without concurrent skilled care. A number of steps need to be taken, therefore, to validate the need for nurse-directed home care and, in particular, the preventive, health teaching, and maintenance aspects of service.

Is nurse-directed service less costly than medically directed home care?

Does it do more than medically directed home care to maintain independence and health?

If these two questions could be answered affirmatively, the recommended policy development would be strengthened greatly.

One research project (Dreher, 1982) found that a nurse responsible for all home health service needs of a given geographical population is much less costly than Medicare reimbursable home care services. Whether this wider range of services (maintenance and prevention) increases health status has not been measured. The studies by Berkman and Syme and by Weissert suggest that a wide range of services does increase health status; however, those analyses did not separate preventive costs from those of curative care.

A useful study could be conducted with two matched populations of elderly receiving home care, one using Dreher's model, which is based on per capita costs of comprehensive nurse-directed care, the other measuring per capita costs of current Medicare reimbursable services, which are physician-directed. Such a study would reveal the costs and outcome of the two types of care and provide the data needed for the first two steps in changing policy: (1) what need will the proposed policy fill and (2) will it increase health?

Incrementalism High in Cost

The third step, a choice between incremental gains or new policy direction, is fairly clear in this instance. Incrementalism already has clouded the issues since simply adding on to the existing medical framework will not provide answers for a comparison between medical- and nurse-directed home care. The DHEW (1979), Berkman and Syme (1979), and Weissert (1980) studies show that preventive and maintenance care are extraordinarily expensive to maintain when added to the medical model rather than when delivered as services without concurrent costly skilled and technological care. New policy is needed to allow the measurement of outcome and cost of only those services deemed necessary by a nurse.

This proposed new policy direction could be difficult to implement because physicians would lose a power base in health care delivery. Although home care is hardly a lucrative venture for physicians (they rarely see patients at home and receive no reimbursement for care delivered by home health agency personnel) they do have the benefit of directing those services. Physicians must provide certificates of eligibility, referral, and orders, without which a Medicare patient will not be accepted for home care. This gatekeeping activity strengthens physicians' overall position as the unquestioned leaders and directors of all health care.

To gain their acceptance of nurse-directed care, or to at least decrease their resistance, physician benefit trade-offs would be required. For example, primary care physicians should be included in every admission of a patient to home care, even if for nonmedical reasons, so that the services given will be as individualized as necessary and as beneficial as possible. Bringing in the physicians as required consultants could take the threat out of their losing direction of care.

To further sweeten the benefit, and to make the consultation more likely to occur, physicians should be paid for the submission of the medical history. A complete medical history obviously is needed as a basis for providing safe and effective care. For example, it is essential to have background information on any chronic diseases such as hypertension or diabetes since their presence can very much influence both the medical and nursing care given for a fractured leg or a concussion or surgery. Preventive and maintenance care such as exercise and nutrition also are influenced by past trauma or surgery and by the presence of chronic disease. Clearly, the complete medical history is required for home care of the elderly, and such data often are inadequate or missing. Eliminating the time spent by the nurse trying to obtain such data, and the cost of inadequate or inappropriate care resulting from a poor data base, could make up for the cost of paying physicians for the needed information.

Goals: Economic and Qualitative

Goals to be achieved by nurse-directed home care services are both economic and qualitative. Costs of crisis care for the elderly under these recommendations could decrease but with concomitant cost increases in preventive or maintenance service. This comparison would need to be made on a per capita basis since the number of elderly is growing and health expenditures in the aggregate therefore would rise even with cost-saving actions. These are long-term goals.

For the short term, this proposed policy might appear not to be cost effective; resources and a new system of delivery of care would need to be developed. Although this eventually could improve the cost effectiveness of services, the initial investment would be costly. Community resources, now geared to illness resolution, with emphasis on care delivery by expensive professionals, would need to be refocused. Priority would have to be given to the development and mobilization of maintenance and preventive services. Fewer professionals would be needed in the service delivery; instead, their expertise would be used as planners, directors, and evaluators.

Assurances to Payers

The seventh and final step in this proposed public policy development would be to assure the payers of high-quality, cost-effective care. Public policy demands outcome measurements that clearly have been absent in the Medicare program. Desired outcomes of a nurse-directed home care program might be:

- a decrease in the percentage of the elderly admitted to institutions
- no increased cost per capita (except for inflationary reasons) in substituting appropriate preventive and maintenance services for medical care.

PROBLEMS WITH PHYSICIAN-DIRECTED CARE

Although physicians now bear the legal responsibility for certifying patients for Medicare home care services, they have, as noted, insufficient contact with the patients during the care process to know what is occurring or what is needed. Nurses essentially have the authority as to when to give care, what to give, and when to discharge the patient. They have little accountability under the present framework for outcomes of care, for cost effectiveness of services, or even for the continuing eligibility of patients. They are expected to recommend to physicians that ineligible patients be discharged but they have no responsibility for certifying continuing eligibility. The isolation of physicians from home care is responsible for many costly and inappropriate services. As it is now, the care ordered often is more technological and more sophisticated than necessary and clearly is geared to resolving problems rather than avoiding them through preventive activities.

In acute care settings such as the hospital, physiotherapy, speech therapy, and occupational therapy are available only during limited hours. At other times, nurses or even aides carry out the prescribed activities. If this is safe and appropriate for acutely ill patients, why does Medicare policy require those services to be delivered by expensive specialists during the less acute, more stable convalescent phase at home?

Nurse's aide services are reimbursable only when supervised by a nurse and only when concurrent with skilled nursing care. The supervision usually is by conference with the aide, not eyes-on direction.

These three caregiver models—nurse-physician, other specialists (physical, occupational, and speech therapists) and nurse's aides—could be modified substantially to promote accountability and cost effectiveness. The physician role of care planner and gatekeeper for eligibility status could be bypassed easily. The plans (or orders) nearly are always modified by nurses and certification of eligibility may be legitimate but rarely stays unchanged for the length of service time Medicare allows (30 days). It might be far more productive to require nurses to certify and monitor eligibility and to have them develop the plans of care. It then would not be as easy to manipulate care for hidden purposes and accountability would be increased. Physicians are important in home care, but not in their current roles. If they saw the patients in the home, the medical care they ordered would tend to be more appropriate and less costly. A number of patients in the author's research study (Chapters 5 and 6) are good examples.

For example, a physician ordered expensive blood and respiratory tests for an emphysema patient to analyze her increased shortness of breath. If the physician could have witnessed her disabilities in maneuvering with hip dysplasia, her smoking between oxygen use, and her lack of personal care services, it would have been apparent that the laboratory studies were unnecessary and irrelevant. Another woman, in liver failure, did not require further medication but did need fluids and laboratory studies.

Instead of costly readmission to the hospital, other patients could have been managed safely at home if the physician had made a visit and evaluated their health status there. In the study, one such patient was a woman in chronic kidney failure, another an elderly man experiencing mild but recurrent transient ischemic attacks. Neither could withstand an office visit in the very cold and icy weather and so were hospitalized for their care.

Another important needed physician role is to provide a comprehensive history of illness to the nurses developing a plan of care. Again, the patients in the research study provided graphic examples of the costly and inadequate care provided when their health history was incomplete. The woman recovering from a broken hip whose diabetes and hypertension were neglected was one example; another was a woman with multiple vision and neuromuscular and cardiovascular impairments who qualified for only eight hours a week of aide service because her only documented medical condition was a leg ulcer.

Physiotherapists, occupational therapists, and speech therapists providing home care usually are unnecessary and costly. If such services can be provided by nurses or by aides when the patient is acutely ill, then during convalescence the care most likely could be provided by nurses or, under nursing direction, by aides or family members. Specialists nearly always need to make a home assessment so that the care ordered uses available resources and is safely planned for; once the plan is made, the services may not need to be delivered by the specialist. Indeed, during convalescence when care increasingly is self-provided, group therapy may be more appropriate than one-to-one. Therefore, exercises and activities could be carried out by nurses and aides during their regularly scheduled visits early in rehabilitation. Later, when patients are more mobile and stable, the services may best be provided in a central place such as in the home health agency office.

Changes in the home health system recommended here would place the nurse in the position of directing services and having accountability for health outcomes and cost effectiveness. Physicians would be required to provide a comprehensive health data base and would act as consultants, in the home, to nurses providing care. Other specialists also would act as consultants and care planners within their disciplines but care would be delivered by nurses during their regularly scheduled visits or by aides under nursing supervision.

REFERENCES

Berkman, L., & Syme, L. Social networks, host resistance, and mortality. *American Journal of Epidemiology*, November 1979, *101*, 186-204.

Clinton, C. *Local success and federal failure*. Cambridge, Mass.: ABT Books, 1979.

Davis, K. *Competition in health care*. Paper presented at the American Public Health Association Convention, Los Angeles, November 1981.

Dreher, M. Unpublished research on community funded nursing, 1982.

Dubos, R. *The mirage of health*. New York: The Macmillan Company, 1959.

Gibson, G. The status of health services research. *Health Service Research*, November 1978, 219-222.

Ginzberg, E. *The limits of health reform*. New York: Basic Books, Inc., 1977.

Home health and other in-home services. Department of Health, Education, and Welfare, Report to Congress, November 1979.

Mechanic, D. *Politics, medicine and society*. New York: John Wiley & Sons, Inc., 1974.

New York State Legislature, Long Term Health Care Program, Chapter 895, 1977.

Pegels, C. *Health care and the elderly*. Rockville, Md.: Aspen Systems Corporation, 1980.

Trager, B. Home health services and health insurance. *Medical Care*, January-February 1971, 89-98.

Vladeck, B. *The design of failure: Health policy and the structure of federalism*. New York: Columbia University Center for Community Health Services, August 1977.

Vladeck, B. *Unloving care*. New York: Basic Books, Inc., 1980.

Weissert, W. *Effects and costs of day care and homemaker services for the chronically ill elderly*. National Center for Health Services Research (NCHSR), February 1980.

Chapter 9

Public Policy's Failure To Meet the Health Needs of the Elderly

The health care needs of the elderly have become one of the greatest sources of concern and one of the major expenses of government. Elderly persons are more likely to become ill than are younger members of the population and are more likely to have chronic or debilitating illness: 40 percent of those over the age of 65 are limited by chronic disease (Callahan, 1980). In addition, health care expenditures have risen faster than other costs and the elderly, living on fixed incomes, are finding a disproportionate amount of their resources going for such services. The elderly population not only is growing in number and percentage of the national population but also is living longer. The net increase on Social Security rolls every year is 600,000. In the next 50 years the total population of the United States is expected to increase by 40 percent while the elderly population doubles (Fox & Clauser, 1980).

This increase in the elderly population has been apparent for years. The growth is especially dramatic when viewed in the context of the society as a whole. Pegels (1980) documents this logarithmic increase: Since 1900 the elderly population has increased 700 percent, the total population 200 percent.

This large group of elderly is experiencing lowered mortality but morbidity, debilitation, and dependence have not decreased proportionately. In a study of home care clients in New York state, half of the Medicare clients had cancer, diabetes, or cardiovascular disease (HSA, 1977).

HIGHEST COST, GREATEST SUBSIDY

Hospital costs are the major outlays for the elderly and they are the health care expenditures most highly subsidized by public funds. Some 88 percent of hospital care for the elderly is paid by government as against only 60 percent of physician care and only 46 percent of all other health services (including home care)

(Pegels, 1980). This division of public financing may reflect the expensiveness of the various categories and the proportionate nonpayment risk to providers when subsidization is lacking.

The division of public dollars for the three types of care (hospital, physician, and other) does not reflect health service needs of the aged, however. What subsidization has done is to further skew care toward acute illness interventions, sophisticated technology, and a life-saving perspective. A quarter of all Medicare dollars was spent on hospital care in the last 12 months of patients' lives (Ginzberg, 1977). Considering that the length of the quality of the life of an aged person in the terminal months usually is not increased in a cost-effective manner by curative medicine, it is reasonable to question the use of expensive technology in the hospital compared to delivering supportive comfort measures in the home. Instead of focusing on current health *cost* problems of the aged, perhaps public policy should take a new direction and strengthen the subsidization of *needed* care. If needed care were available, and paid for, the high amount of inappropriate hospital utilization could well decrease. As it is now, elderly persons who experience a period of weakness, instability, or minor illness that precludes living independently for a while, have only two choices: self-pay for support services in their (or their families') homes or enter a hospital for which public dollars will pay.

Even nursing homes will not be paid by Medicare unless there is a need for skilled care—and if there is, the patients probably can gain reimbursable access to a hospital instead. Although their rates are very high, hospitals are necessary for lifesaving, restorative care. Sometimes hospital care is first priority for the elderly. Surgery, acute crises, and trauma may all require a hospital stay. But utilizing hospitals for chronic care is wasteful of public dollars, of the facilities' resources, and of the aged persons' limited time to enjoy life among family and community. The isolation that hospitals impose could be called unethical when the same public dollars could be spent on less costly services that could increase the quality of life of the elderly. Not only has there been inadequate public payment for needed noninstitutional services, there also has been inadequate development of capacity to provide them, thereby further limiting their use.

A transfer of public funding from institutional medical services to noninstitutional support could be seen as a move to deprive the elderly of lifesaving services. The public must face this issue: is money best used to provide expensive life support services (kidney dialysis, respirators, etc.) to the elderly for whom little or no improvement is possible? Since these resources are finite, is there a priority population for this kind of service delivery, and does the priority grouping exclude the elderly?

As the total population increases in average age, the needs of the elderly may be seen more clearly than when they composed such a small group. Many of the elderly may have a strong preference for support and comfort services. For the same dollar amount a year, a full-time homemaker may be preferable to intermittent five-day hospitalizations for weak, unstable older persons living alone. If they are to depend on public dollars for health care now, they have no choice but to do the best they can for themselves until such time as they become weak or unstable enough to qualify for a few days' hospitalization, which may give them the boost (nutritionally and otherwise) to try again to make it at home alone.

ISSUES BOTH ETHICAL AND ECONOMIC

Policy should address these issues through determination of eligibility for publicly funded care and by decisions to develop new kinds of services. The issues in formulating that policy are ethical as well as economic and, again, professionals have an enormous responsibility to provide data for the public in determining how the nation will care for its aged.

The elderly have little choice in the kind of care they receive unless they are wealthy or very poor. Eligibility for hospital or home care is firmly limited to those in need of acute medical services. Although this makes a good deal of sense for hospitalization, it makes no sense for home care. Nursing home care under Medicare also requires that the patients have acute medical care needs. If the elderly are poor enough to qualify for Medicaid, nursing home care is available for nonmedical maintenance care. But this type of care is rarely the choice of the patient; for some, it is care of last resort. Home care for the poor under Medicaid may or may not include personal support measures; this depends on the state or city of residence. Homemakers are available for self-pay patients but the cost is prohibitive for those without substantial dollar resources.

The percentage of the gross national product (GNP) expended for health care was 10.4 percent in 1982. Not measured in the GNP is the value of family care, especially important for the elderly and disabled. Family care may be the most threatened resource for the elderly. A federal study in 1977 concluded that "the true costs of maintaining the elderly and sick in their own homes have been largely hidden because the greatest portion of such costs represent the services provided by families and friends rather than those provided at public expense" (DHEW, 1977).

Of the disabled elderly, 70 percent live with others; for every disabled person in a nursing home there are two equally disabled living at home (HCA, 1979). Although more than two-thirds of the elderly have family assistance, 90 percent need it. This figure of 20 percent of the elderly without family assistance is bound to increase. The demographic and economic changes the nation has experienced in recent years threaten the existence of family support for the elderly. Once children are independent (and often before), a typical couple becomes a family of two-wage earners. The advent of an aged parent, requiring assistance and supervision, would require one of the wage earners to give up a job to stay home and provide care or the couple would have to pay for a helper to come in. Neither of these choices is economically feasible for most families. Nursing home care, especially if the elderly person can qualify for Medicaid, becomes the solution for many.

THE LONGER LIFE FACTOR

For other families, the geographical distances now common between the elderly and their children make it less likely that the latter can be available to help. Furthermore, as the elderly live longer, their children also are aging; a 65-year-old person is likely to have children in their forties but an 85 year-old may have children who also are aged and disabled. National policy therefore must address the changing nature of families and their resources as well as of the elderly population.

The health sciences, the environment, and other factors have led to longer life spans but the point at which dependency and disability begin has not changed significantly. The needs of the elderly are growing even faster than their numbers so the decline of family assistance is a critical concern.

Research on home health needs of the elderly says their requirements are care for chronic conditions and support for their lessening independence (Callahan, 1980; Kane & Kane, 1978). An argument against the aims of Medicare was that it was "an effort to force chronic care needs into an acute care framework" (Trager, 1971). Functional status has been shown to be the best determinant of the need for home care and of length of service; the lower the functional ability, the higher the need for home care and the longer the service (HSA, 1977).

A separate study by the Home Care Association of New York State (1979) corroborates these findings and also showed that half the over-65 clients in New York State on home care had physical disabilities. A statement by the National League for Nursing at a Congressional hearing on health insurance (NLN, 1980) called for changing the determinants for home care from medical diagnoses to functional status. Ricker-Smith and Trager (1978) note that the chronically ill and elderly have multiple medical diagnoses and that the most recent one (usually crisis oriented) may have no relationship to the need for home care.

Another study reports that only 15 percent of the elderly in need of home care are receiving it (DHEW, 1977). Another 2.3 million need those services and do not have them because of inadequate availability and restrictive eligibility. Other studies show that the needs of the elderly (now as in pre-Medicare years) are for custodial care and a family environment (Feder, 1977; Ginzberg, 1977; Trager, 1971). These last two factors are becoming increasingly important as the population eligible for Medicare increases in number and in average age and as family structure becomes less able to support extra elderly members.

Another study of the elderly demonstrates that the kind of service needed (e.g., skilled vs. custodial) is the best determinant of level of care (institution vs. the patient's home) (HCA, 1979). Furthermore, the medical diagnosis is regarded as not as good an indicator of level of care required as is the need for skilled services.

Although these research findings are consistent, the relationship between needs and Medicare coverage never has been complementary, and never was meant to be. The Medicare statute focuses on home health care as a secondary service, not as a primary one. It reimburses home health service only as a less expensive alternative to hospital care.

Two studies describe patients receiving Medicare home health services and characteristics such as age, sex, living arrangements, and types and number of current medical diagnoses (DHEW, 1979; HCA, 1979). These reports show that the majority of the elderly over 65 (80 percent) have at least one chronic illness, that two-thirds of home care patients are women, and an increasing number of all home care patients (one-third) live alone.

SIX CATEGORIES OF NEEDS

It is apparent that the home health needs of the elderly fall into six categories (each of these is discussed next in more detail):

1. *Chronic illness and/or disability care.* The three major diagnoses of home care clients (cancer, diabetes, cardiovascular disease) all are of a chronic, degenerative, and disabling nature. They require social services, nursing care, nutrition, and personal aid that are of more critical importance than medical care (Munger, 1975).

Cancer often is progressive and fatal. For the elderly, cancer often progresses more slowly and, therefore, leads to a longer period when home care, as opposed to acute care in an institution, is required. The elderly are less able to withstand drastic surgery or the devastating courses of radiation or chemotherapy that may spell cure for younger, more vigorous cancer patients. Instead, the elderly victims often remain at home, receiving palliative and less risky curative measures.

Adult onset diabetes is primarily a disease of middle and old age. Although dietary and medication therapy can maintain blood sugar levels in a normal range, the cellular changes associated with the disease lead to progressive pathology and disability: kidney failure, premature arteriosclerosis and atherosclerosis, higher incidence of heart attacks, vision loss, peripheral vascular insufficiency, and neurological deficits. All of these changes are predictable sequellae of diabetes and lead to the need for further support for patients so they may remain independent in their homes.

Very few medical therapies can delay or prevent the diabetic complications. Retinal surgery and amputations of inadequately perfused toes (or even a leg) are common medical interventions but the most useful therapies are nutrition education, skin care, exercise, foot care, and regular health assessment to identify problems early. These all are nursing skills.

Cardiovascular disease is a "natural" product of aging. The best therapies to prevent crises and further disability are nutrition, weight control, regular exercise and elimination of smoking. These all clearly are within the direction of a nurse. Medication to lower blood pressure or "blood thinners" have been losing favor, with self-care regimes apparently more helpful.

> 2. *Social networks.* Clients remaining in their own homes for care, and those maintaining social ties in the community, both show reduced mortality when compared to matched cohorts receiving similar care in institutions or in relative social isolation. (Berkman & Syme, 1979; Weissert, 1980)

Social networks appear to promote less illness and a longer life than when persons are institutionalized for care. Research has long demonstrated that institutionalized patients tend to become disoriented and depressed. When the elderly live longer, they tend to cost society more money; Social Security benefits, such as pensions and Medicare, have no upper age limitations. Weissert (1979) shows that the elderly maintained at home with support services not only live longer and are happier but also use more services (including institutionalization and outpatient care) than the elderly without home care supports—another indication of increased cost to society. If increased home care, with social supports, would be more costly, would Americans be willing to fund it? How does society value the life of an elderly person? Even before such answers are solicited in making policy decisions, important observations need to be made.

Support systems for the elderly at home have been measured and costed as an additive service. Instead of continuing to maintain the existing health care system, with its expensive emphasis on crisis service, restructuring may be required to meet the needs of today and tomorrow.

Perhaps it would be wise to listen more closely to the elderly. With limited resources a certainty, they may prefer $10,000 of support services in the home to $10,000 of institutional care promised for the last few days or weeks of their lives.

> 3. *Sheltered or congregate housing.* Clients receiving "family type" assistance are more satisfied and less often institutionalized (Kane & Kane, 1978; Kurowski, 1979). With fewer old people having access to assistance from their families, and with more individuals living to old age, this type of living arrangement serves an important need.

Sheltered or congregate housing arrangements provide semi-independent living for the elderly who need minor supervision or assistance with their daily activities. In sheltered housing, assistance is readily available: a nurse on the premises, or a support system of dining services, or resident persons who can help the elderly get out to shopping centers or medical appointments. Congregate housing provides group living for the essentially independent elderly. They may or may not have support services available. They may reside interdependently in single living units, or in a joint setting such as private bedrooms with shared social and dining rooms. Usually security and medical on-call arrangements are provided.

As single persons or couples reach old age, their economic and social resources become depleted although their physical and mental capacities still support their independence. Congregate housing provides for that independence to continue safely and satisfactorily.

Without the availability of such living arrangements, the elderly, especially those alone, find nursing homes or isolated welfare housing the only options as they become poor and infirm. Since these two options almost always are paid for by public funds, it would make social and economic sense for government to support congregate and sheltered housing at least in part; the daily cost per resident surely could be less than institutional (nursing home) care.

4. *Personal services.* A major percentage of the aged receiving skilled home care or confined to institutions would live independently if personal services such as meal preparation, shopping, laundry, bathing were available (Gary, 1979; Kane, 1978).

When the elderly lose the ability to provide these personal services for themselves, a number of changes occur—all of them unsatisfactory to the older people, their families, and the public payer. If the family is willing and able, the elderly person needing help with day to day activities moves in with them. If there is no family resource, the elderly rely on each other but this arrangement is unstable and predictably unreliable and short term.

Elderly persons who own their own homes, or who have savings in the bank, are not eligible for publicly funded support services such as Medicaid offers for the poor. Medicare provides limited, short-term support services if an acute medical need is concurrent but that eligibility ceases when the need for skilled care ends. Elderly persons with property or savings must "spend down" (deplete these resources), paying for their own support services until they reach the economic level of the poor before they can receive subsidized support services in the home. Of course, by then they no longer may have a home. Requiring the independent and economically stable elderly to become dependent if they are to receive assistance is a financially foolish and socially questionable policy.

Nursing homes are as expensive as they are because they must be staffed for the 24-hour care needed by some of the residents; many residing there, however, require only intermittent and relatively inexpensive support services. However, because those services are not available anywhere else (unless through self-pay) even the mildly infirm must be cared for at high public expense.

5. *Payment for drugs, eyeglasses, preventive podiatry, and dentistry.* These health-promoting and maintenance (and curative) services probably are cost-effective investments for the elderly since they strengthen these individuals' independence and safety.

In the home health agency where this research was conducted, the patient population was increasingly reflecting accidents as the reason for home care services—20 percent of those in the study. Previously, illness had been the overwhelming cause for referral for care. Correct eyeglasses alone may be able to prevent falls or cooking injuries. Inability to pay for drugs can have disastrous implications for hypertensive patients (strokes), for glaucoma patients (blindness), for arthritics (falls or becoming bedridden). Anti-inflammatory drugs for arthritics are particularly expensive, with $40 a month a not uncommon cost. Any of these predictable undesirable outcomes that would result without the drug therapy can cause expensive institutionalization that clearly would cost more than the preventive or maintenance care.

6. *Day care.* Families willing and able to assist and monitor their elderly members in the evening and at night often cannot be available for daytime care. In addition, the mental health of all family members is enhanced if the elderly can participate in an organized program away from home base. Day care may make the difference between independence and institutionalization.

In more and more families, all the adult members are in the work force. Much more rarely is the woman home and unemployed after her children are grown. Usually the children reach independence at the very time grandparents are becoming more dependent but the family resource no longer is available to those elderly in the person of a daughter or daughter-in-law who stays at home.

Elderly patients frequently are quite independent physically—they can walk and bathe and care for themselves—but because of predictable frailty (poor eyesight, arthritis, poor balance) may not be entirely safe unattended for long hours. Mental state, as well, can influence forgetfulness; mild disorientations may appear only rarely but can put the elderly at risk for injury when they occur.

For these reasons a day care center, which offers safety supervision as well as social interactions, allows families to continue to care for their elderly at home.

Day care, like drugs, eyeglasses, preventive care, and personal support services, can decrease expensive institutionalization. Existing policy covers only the crisis care often caused by the absence of such preventive services. The shortsighted penny-wise and pound-foolish approach continues to be overly costly and deeply unsatisfying to the nation's elderly.

The health needs of the aged primarily involve assistance in self-care on a daily basis. Institutionalization is a predictable occurrence for acute illness or extended care; it also is the result of the failure to supply adequate supportive and preventive care. In focusing on the major cost problems of the elderly (hospital and physician care) Medicare legislation has ignored the major health needs in determining benefits. Meeting these health maintenance needs might decrease substantially the payment needed for restorative services.

OTHER MAJOR LEGISLATION

While Medicare is aimed primarily at payment of the hospital and supplemental costs of acute care for the elderly, other federal legislation has targeted their social and health-related needs.

Medicaid: Title XIX of the Social Security Act (P.L. 89-97)

Medicaid was passed with Medicare in 1965. It is a program to deliver health and health-related services to the medically indigent. Previously, welfare funds had assisted in the payment of health care bills for the poor. Under Medicaid those same poor people are covered and each individual state decides whether to broaden eligibility to include those whose income places them above the welfare cut-off level but who, because of extensive medical bills, will need public assistance. These are the medically indigent.

Medicaid funds are part federal and part state. The federal contribution is at least 50 percent and may rise as high as 77 percent. The federal contribution is inversely related to the average per capita income in each state. The state determines eligibility criteria and the scope of reimbursable services, as long as they cover at least the minimum required. Most states chose to cover only individuals previously eligible for welfare.

This legislation determined a federal floor for services but not a ceiling. In addition, it committed the federal government to pay half or three-quarters of costs that states could decide unilaterally to incur for the program. Not only have costs risen dramatically, but the federal government has had little control over limiting them.

Unlike Medicare, clients under Medicaid do not have to be homebound or need skilled care in order to receive home health services. They do, however, still need physician certification for care. Home services do not have to be delivered through a certified home health agency (except where one is available). Medicaid pays for personal services where the states decide to include them. Payment rates for most services are somewhat lower than Medicare. The elderly or disabled poor are eligible for Medicare benefits and the extra Medicaid services (long-term home health care, personal services). A smaller percentage of total program expenditures goes to home health services but more absolute dollars than in Medicare.

Federal-State Social Service Programs: Title XX, 1975

This amendment to the Social Security Act provides grants-in-aid to states so they can make available certain needed social services, including personal care, home health aides, and home care. Physician direction of care is not required but social service professional direction is. States pay 25 percent of funds that are federally disbursed on the basis of population.

Federal expenditures under Medicaid are determined to a large extent by individual states' decisions on provision of benefits; under Title XX, however, they have a ceiling that is set annually. The states can make Medicaid an entitlement program but still have flexibility and control over which services to offer; the federal government must help pay for those state-determined services.

Older Americans Act: 1965 (P.L. 89-73)

This federal program partially funds services to keep the elderly independent. Grants-in-aid are made to the states for home health services, including personal care. Also allowed are funds for residential repairs and transportation.

The funds are targeted for a variety of programs, depending on the priorities in any given state; may or may not provide the needed social services for the elderly; and vary from state to state. Medicare is the only truly federal health program and it is for acute medical problems. There is no similar federal program for the elderly that assures nationwide eligibility and access for supportive health services.

One of the more troubling aspects of regional or state programs is that they exist in such isolated splendor that they are potentially short-lived; beneficiaries are attracted from a wider area than can be served; and as the trade-offs become apparent, the very existence of the effort is threatened because it draws resources away from other areas. This is a particular problem when the competing programs provide more immediate and visible benefits, such as new roads or more police.

The Medicaid program in New York City is an example. Not only did potential beneficiaries flock to that city, which covered care in such generous ways, but New York soon began to weigh its financial share in the expensive program against other needed municipal services, such as transportation and safety. Even though the city's Medicaid program appears unusually beneficial to recipients, demographic data can partially support the broader increase in services; the program is not all that out of line with needs. There are more elderly living alone in need of medical attendants in New York City than in other parts of the state or country (HSA, 1977). The city, as do all governmental entities, looks at a program in terms of (1) whether it is meeting a need and (2) what alternate services those committed dollars could buy. An isolated regional program, even a good one, loses some credibility and value simply because it is not broad enough and lacks widespread support, and because the dollars invested could be used for so many other projects.

Care for the elderly therefore can depend more on local resources than on the individuals' needs. Regional programs suffer in stability because they are more vulnerable to loss of funding resulting from only minor changes in needs or priorities. National programs and priorities not only do not shift as easily but also are more likely to recognize the needs of the disadvantaged.

The political weaknesses in regional or local programs (which tend to respond to more visible short-term goals) provide a strong argument for a federal program for health services for the elderly. Regional programs not only tend to be more unstable (because of easily shifted funding) but also can promote inequities in service availability. A national policy requiring certain supportive health services could help assure equity, access, and quality.

Regions and localities develop the specific services in ways they say would best benefit their elderly. New York City might choose to continue the home attendant program, whereas Fargo, N.D., might opt for transportation services, or another community might choose to fund nutritional services. Under a policy of certain required minimum services, each locality receiving federal funds would be accountable for providing care that would keep the elderly independent, healthy, and out of institutions. This would be consistent with the aims of Medicare but the process would become far more flexible.

The desires of the elderly remain the same: a long, healthy life, independence, and the opportunity to remain in their own community. If they are to achieve all this, more than acute or convalescent medical care services will be required. The challenge is for development of a policy that meets the needs of the elderly in a cost-effective manner acceptable to all of society.

REFERENCES

Berkman, L., & Syme, S. Social networks, host resistance, and mortality. *American Journal of Epidemiology*, November 1979, *109*.

Callahan, J. Responsibility of families for their severely disabled elders. *Health Care Financing Review*, Winter 1980, 29-48.

Feder, J. Medicare implementation and the policy process. *Journal of Health Policy, Politics & Law*, Summer 1977, 173-189.

Fox, P., & Clauser, S. Trends in nursing home expenditures: Implications for aging policy. *Health Care Financing Review*, Fall 1980, 65-70.

Gary, L.R. *Home health care regulation: Issues and opportunities*. New York: Hunter College, 1979.

Ginzberg, E. *The limits of health reform*. New York: Basic Books, Inc., 1977.

Home care in New York state. Albany, N.Y.: Home Care Association of New York State, May 1979.

Home health: The need for a national policy to better provide for the elderly. Department of Health, Education, and Welfare, Report to Congress, December 1977.

Home health and other in-home services. Department of Health, Education, and Welfare, DHEW Report to Congress, November 1979.

Home health care: Its utilization, costs and reimbursement. New York: Health Services Agency of New York City, November 1977.

Kane, R., & Kane, R. Care of the aged—An old problem in search of new solutions. *Science*, May 26, 1978, 913-918.

Kurowski, B. *Cost per episode of home health care: Executive summary*. Boulder, Colo.: University of Colorado, CHSR, March 1979.

Munger, P. Medicare and Medicaid: The failure of the present health care system for the elderly. *Arizona Law Review*, 1975, *17*.

National League of Nursing. Statement on home care presented to the U.S. Congress, House Ways and Means Subcommittee on Health's hearings on health insurance, February 12, 1980.

Pegels, C. *Health care and the elderly*. Rockville, Md.: Aspen Systems Corporation, 1980.

Ricker-Smith, K., & Trager, B. In-home health services in California. *Medical Care*, March 1978.

Trager, B. Home health services and health insurance. *Medical Care*, January-February 1971, 89-98.

Weissert, W. *Effects and costs of day care and homemaker services for the chronically ill elderly*. National Center for Health Services Research (NCHSR), February 1980.

Chapter 10

Public Accountability and Care of the Elderly

Grow old along with me!
The best is yet to be,
The last of life, for which the first was made.

Robert Browning, "Rabbi Ben Ezra" (1864)

Although the intent of Medicare policy has always been to substitute home services for convalescent care in an institution, the process of providing those services has resulted in the provision of costly and inappropriate medical care. The system was destined for change, in part because costs had become so high and in part because the needs of the elderly were not being met. Those unmet needs inevitably would become even more urgent as the numbers of elderly grew and as their important resource—family assistance—became less available.

Hospitalization probably will always be the most expensive care option, so the intent of Medicare home health services is valid and increasingly valued. The ways of fulfilling that intent will change over the years, however, for the kinds of care needed and resources available demand it.

Recommendations for change in this chapter are intended to promote cost containment and to develop a system that will help meet the health needs of the elderly. The recommendations are based on the expectation that home care services can decrease institutionalization of the elderly by preventing crises before they occur, by maintaining health at optimum levels, and by promoting health through more effective self-care, compliance, and safety awareness (Pegels, 1980; Trager, 1980; Van Dyke & Brown, 1972).

The recommendations are made with the knowledge that health policy has entered an era where cost containment is of primary importance. An analysis of the role of quality of care assessment in the 1980s describes the current motive in such evaluation as "protective," i.e., "attempting to prevent a level of cuts in services

179

that would push the quality of care below some extremely minimal level.'' In the past, quality was addressed as "enhancing," which meant to maximize health regardless of costs (Brook & Lohr, 1981). The recommendations here are made in the more defensive, or "protective," framework while still supporting experimental changes in the process of home health services delivery that could increase quality and still contain costs.

THE RECOMMENDED NEW CRITERIA

Medicare now requires that patients meet certain criteria in order to receive home care services. It is recommended that home care services be limited to those who otherwise would be institutionalized, that criteria be developed to assure valid eligibility, and that custodial services be allowed if they are needed and are cost effective in preventing institutionalization. It also is proposed that outcome measurements be made after a specified time to ascertain whether the service provided was successful and whether the patient still is at risk for institutionalization or no longer qualifies for home care. These recommendations would require major changes in the three current eligibility criteria and would:

1. Abolish "homebound" status and substitute two other eligibility criteria:
   a. that a need for home adaptation of required care be demonstrated.
   b. that functional status and living arrangement (alone or with family) be the basis for determining eligibility for additional services.
2. Replace the "skilled care" criterion with reimbursement for only those services required to prevent, or substitute for, institutionalization, including provisions for at least one of the following:
   a. that medically directed curative (nursing) care, such as medications, complex dressings, or treatments, be supplied when required for an existing condition.
   b. that professional nursing intervention (teaching, counseling, and health maintenance) for patient and/or family be provided.
   c. that ancillary services (homemaker, home health aide) based on the patient's DMS-1 rating be provided. (The Determination of Medical Standards (DMS-1) scale was developed by the New York State Health Department Bureau of Research and Evaluation to evaluate patients' placement in long-term care facilities. It is a numerical summary of self-care impairments, mental status, and nursing services needed.)
3. Replace "physician-established plan of care" with the following requirements:
   a. that a complete medical history be provided by the regular medical caregiver.

b. that a new nurse-established plan for nursing care be cosigned by the physician if care is for a medical condition.

"Homebound" status should be eliminated for three reasons:

1. because it is easily manipulated (nearly 40 percent of the research study population were not homebound)
2. because it may actually increase services delivered by encouraging the manifestation of skilled care needs in the permanently homebound so they can meet the dual criteria for home care eligibility.
3. because it may be focusing care on the very population the law intended to omit from coverage—the chronically ill elderly in need of custodial care.

As to the first of the proposed new criteria to replace "homebound," if patients require care in their residence, it obviously must be adapted to their resources, abilities, and family's support. This care may include teaching, demonstration, problem solving with the patients to accommodate their preferences, and counseling to help them assume a successful self-care routine.

As for the second part of that recommendation, functional status and living arrangement, the author's research study demonstrated that nurses provided extended services to patients who lived alone and who were functionally in need of assistance, so those elements should be made formal parts of the home care structure. Professional services such as teaching, counseling, and health maintenance may be necessary because of the patients' debility or because they have no family. Custodial care may be needed for either of those same reasons. The two together (living alone and a functional disability) may require home-based care of a professional nurse as well as homemaker assistance.

Although a full complement of skilled and custodial care can maintain many patients at home instead of in an institution, the services required for some may be so extensive that they may be costlier than in an institution or in an outpatient facility. If this is the case, public dollars should be expended only to the amount that would have been paid for the patient to receive care in the less expensive setting.

REASONS FOR CHANGE

There are three major reasons why the skilled care criterion should be changed:

1. Nurses interpret it broadly so they can provide comprehensive preventive care; nearly a third of the patients in the research study were receiving home health services although their need for skilled care no longer was apparent.

2. Medically curative services for an acute episode cannot be isolated from care needed for chronic conditions, as the study demonstrated.
3. Home health services have not cut the overall costs of an episode of illness but there are indications that preventive and maintenance care may be able to lower overall costs of the elderly (Callahan, 1980; DHEW, 1977; Hammond, 1979).

All of these would initiate major changes: these would erase the requirement for a medical episode in order to qualify patients for services and would make a much wider scope of services available to them once admitted to care. The rationale for these apparently costly changes is that preventive or maintenance care in the home for the elderly may be cost effective. The cost of six home care nursing visits (1983 data) is approximately the same as one day of hospitalization in the study area ($300). Professional nursing care aimed at prevention and maintenance can accomplish a great deal in six separate hours of service, and very few of the elderly were hospitalized for only one day. Ancillary care can go even further: four hours a day of home health aide services is only $324 for a seven-day week of service, again about equal to one day in a hospital.

The most obvious question is: "Wouldn't this liberalization mean that everyone over 65 could have daily household assistance?" The answer is that services must be justified as necessary to prevent institutionalization. It is recommended that care components be allowable based on their contribution to keeping the individual out of an institution. Documentation would be required to justify each service as needed for that purpose.

CONTROL OF CARE

The third qualifying criterion in the Medicare statute—requiring that a physician establish the plan for home care services—has proved to be wasteful of resources and inadequate for the provision of needed care. As was discussed earlier, because physicians rarely if ever participate in the delivery of health services in the home, they are ill-equipped to know what ones are needed. The continuum of care from the institution depends very much on the resources available in the home—and physicians generally are unaware of what is, or is not, available there. Nurses give or supervise the majority of home care and are especially knowledgeable about promoting self-care and adapting home and family resources to the patients' needs. Nursing is autonomous in these nonmedical areas and physicians are not skilled or knowledgeable to provide those professional nursing services. That also would be a negation of nurses' accountability. This split responsibility can result in neither professional's acknowledging accountability to provide needed comprehensive care.

Physician plans of care are wasteful of resources because they focus on the medical components of treatment, regardless of need. Medical services are the most expensive available and physicians, trained in the detection and cure of disease and pathology, use them almost exclusively. However, service in the home is meant to be assisted self-care and has little relationship to treatment needed for the acute stage of an illness.

In the research study, half of the physician plans of care were found to be inadequate even for the limited medical aspects of care. To meet the comprehensive needs of patients, all of these physician plans were revised by the nurses providing care. The physician plans often omitted information that had a critical impact on nursing care to be delivered. For instance, nearly a third of the patients who were known diabetics were not identified as such on the physician's referral or plan of care.

The data from the research study indicate that primary care physicians wrote more adequate plans than did specialists and provided more comprehensive data on primary diagnoses than for secondary diagnoses. These findings indicate that the medical data base often is sparse and inadequate for the effective care of elderly in the home. By requiring a more complete referral, and by charging the practitioners who usually oversee the patients' health care with that duty, the data base could become more adequate and the ensuing care be more complete. All of this would shift the accountability and direction of nursing care, placing both where they legitimately belong—with the nurse.

Nursing Care Reimbursement

Medically directed nursing care, the only kind allowable under Medicare, would continue to be reimbursed under the recommended framework. Every referral received by the home health agency would be evaluated by a nurse. If criteria for institutional prevention services were met, a plan would be developed by the nurse and submitted to the patient's primary care provider for additional information regarding the individual's medical condition(s). In this way, nursing care required for medical conditions would be assured even when the primary reason for service might be nonmedical.

For example, a patient might be referred for ADL (activities of daily living) assessment and strengthening, and information on any existing arthritis or vision problems would be helpful. Patients also could be referred for nonmedical service such as short-term custodial care during a family's absence or for counseling and the establishment of a healthful dietary and exercise regime after the deep depression and self-neglect following the death of a spouse.

Under existing guidelines, as noted in earlier chapters, medically directed care is required in order to provide access to other needed service. Reimbursable nursing care is available in only one place—in the home—and only when it is medically directed for the express purpose of resolving the current medical condition. Nursing services in institutions are not reimbursed separately but are built into the aggregate costs of services, which also include housekeeping, dietary, and fuel expenses.

Nursing services in outpatient clinics or HMOs traditionally are part of overall service charges as well, so there is no identifiable paid unit of nursing care for clients anywhere but in the home. Nurse practitioners in outpatient practice are receiving fee-for-service payment and Medicare will reimburse their work in areas certifiably underserved by physicians (P.L. 95-210, the Rural Health Clinic Services Act of 1977, the Medicare and Medicaid Amendments), but the services are reimbursed as a substitution for medical care, not as nursing care.

The research study demonstrated that patients could avoid institutionalization through the use of professional nursing services other than medically curative ones. Teaching, counseling, and health maintenance are useful in preventing institutionalization; thus it is recommended that those services be identified and reimbursed as free-standing, independent units.

Ancillary Service Needs

The use of ancillary services could be determined by the patients' functional disabilities and living arrangement. Those living alone would be eligible for some of the assistance usually provided by families, such as homemaker services. Those functionally disabled or in need of frequent care would be eligible for additional support services such as nighttime "sitters" or additional hours of home health aide services.

An objective and already developed mechanism, the DMS-1 form could be used in making allotments of extra services. Patients with higher dependency scores would be eligible for more services. Data on nursing home patients indicate that many do not need the level of care being paid for in the institution but could function well at home with added services. The cost for that comprehensive home service still could be lower than nursing home care. A 1979 survey (HCA, 1979) showed that 22 percent of the patients on home care in New York state had DMS-1 scores in the range that would have qualified them for a skilled nursing facility (nursing home). The availability of custodial services may be more important than disability level when the choice is made between home care and nursing home.

Nursing Home without Walls

It is recommended that Medicare adopt the Nursing Home without Walls concept (NYS, 1980). If Medicare were to adopt a similar trade-off between home and institutional care, its limitations on custodial services would have to be relaxed since those would be the ones needed to prevent institutionalization. Under existing law, Medicare pays only for intermittent skilled care in the home, or for nursing home care if the patient has skilled-care needs.

Often, all that is needed to maintain a person at home is mild supervision or assistance with meals or dressing. These regular but simple needs cannot be met economically by multiple home visits each day. The elderly in need of such assistance might do well in congregate housing (as discussed in Chapter 9). An example of that type of facility would have numerous private rooms for individuals or couples who would live fairly independently with assistance and supervision available from resident custodial personnel and a resident health professional. In some instances a public health nurse would make a regular daily visit to each senior citizen housing center and could see up to 15 or 20 chronically ill or disabled elderly in one morning, whereas individual visits could be made to only two or three private homes in the same time. Either plan is less costly than admitting those elderly persons to nursing homes.

Although nearly all of the elderly would prefer to remain in their own homes, the public subsidization needed to accomplish the necessary safety and support services may become prohibitive. Rather than limiting care to expensive skilled treatment in the home or in an institution, other services and other settings could be developed that would be more attractive to the elderly and be less costly to the public. Congregate or sheltered housing are possibilities. Other proposals are discussed later.

Studies on the use of custodial and support services show that they increase overall cost of home care and the use of other services, such as hospitalization (Berkman & Syme, 1979; Weissert, 1980). Recommendations to increase the utilization of support services, therefore, are tied to using them instead of, not in conjunction with, expensive skilled or medically oriented care.

REIMBURSEMENT STRUCTURE REVISIONS

A number of changes also are recommended in the reimbursement structure. Reimbursement regulations now have no incentives for cost saving. Rather than paying full cost per service, it is recommended that reimbursement be based on the national average expenditure for a given episode of care with fee-for-service repayment eliminated. This would mean that providers in underserved and lower cost areas would receive higher than usual reimbursement and those in overserved and higher cost areas would get lower than usual recompense. This might serve to decrease the maldistribution of providers somewhat. It also would allow for discretion in types of services provided.

The model for this proposal is the DRG program (diagnosis-related groups), in which reimbursement to hospitals is based on their average cost of caring for a person of a given age, with a given medical diagnosis, and with given functional disabilities. Prospective reimbursement for hospital payment for Medicare patients was passed into law in the Reconciliation Act of 1982. The regulations were developed in 1983 for nationwide Medicare reimbursement. Although Medicare long-term care (including home health) was omitted from prospective reimbursement, there are plans to include home health later. For a DRG proposal for home care, the diagnoses used should be secondary, not primary. The reason is that by the time patients can be cared for at home rather than in an institution, it is not the medical diagnosis that determines that need but the impact of that diagnosis.

For example, a patient with an acute myocardial infarction might require expensive in-hospital services, including technological assessment and monitoring, a specialized intensive care unit, and extensive laboratory tests. The DRG reimbursement would be high. Another patient might be hospitalized with a back injury that required traction and bed rest but no expensive sophisticated services, so the hospital DRG reimbursement would be considerably lower. However, when each patient is discharged, the home health needs would be similar—both would need assistance with self-care until their strength returned. Therefore, home health care reimbursement should be based on functional status and living arrangement. The different medical diagnoses may be of little value in predicting the cost of home care but the other criteria will be. Patients living alone require more services than those living with family members.

Nursing Diagnoses

The secondary diagnoses that would be most useful in this reimbursement scheme are nursing diagnoses. These are statements of actual or potential health deficits and may or may not be related to any disease process. They spell out what the health deficit is, what the related cause may be, and include statements on functional disabilities. Typical nursing diagnoses for the elderly might identify:

- an inability to feed or dress self related to arthritis deformities of both hands
- malnourishment and weakness related to depression over death of spouse.

These not only pinpoint a health status that can be improved but also suggest the most appropriate therapy or support by naming the cause of the problem (Mundinger, 1980; Mundinger & Jauron, 1975). Nursing diagnoses are particularly helpful in planning home services because they focus on self-care potential and states of health that are not necessarily related to medical problems. The resolution of these health deficits (or nursing diagnoses) may lead to independent living once again for the elderly. Because they are the focus of cost-effective home care, these nursing diagnoses constitute an excellent method of determining reimbursement potential.

Outcome Evaluations

When nursing diagnoses and family type resources are used as criteria for receiving home care, outcome evaluations become the logical and accountable method of assessing the ultimate value of services. Reimbursement based on achievement of prospectively determined outcomes has been recommended for some time (Kane & Kane, 1978; Levenson, 1979; Van Dyke, 1972). The outcomes for care of the elderly can be measured by the traditional health status indexes such as improved health or return to work, but that method often is a problem for the aged population. The great majority of the elderly (most estimates are 75 percent over the age of 65) have at least one chronic disease and few will get any better or will be able to increase productivity as a result of care provided. A far more sensitive indicator of effective care for the chronically ill, such as the elderly, is the measurement of unmet needs (Carr, 1980; Wolfe, 1977, 1980). In this framework, care deficits for appropriate treatment of health problems are identified and the outcomes are measured by the effectiveness of care in meeting those deficits.

HOME CARE BENEFICIARIES

There are two distinct populations of elderly who can benefit from home care so two sets of outcome criteria are appropriate:

1. those who have been hospitalized with an acute episode of illness or disability and subsequently require convalescent health care outside the institution
2. those who have not been institutionalized but are at risk for such placement because of their deteriorating health or waning self-care abilities.

For the first group, some degree of cure or rehabilitation may be possible. The outcome of home services therefore can be the desired health status. For example, a patient recovering from a fractured hip might have these health outcomes:

1. ambulates independently using crutches
2. ambulates independently without assistive devices
3. assumes self-care, including bathing and cooking.

Each of these outcomes, or goals, would be planned with an achievement date. As those dates were reached, an evaluative report would be made to the reimbursement agency. Discharge from home care services would be determined by the date on which the patient had achieved the health status of again being safely self-sufficient. Members of the second group now have no access to reimbursable services, yet by neglecting their at-risk status they are certain candidates for crisis illness or accident care that then will result in eligibility for expensive rehabilitative care.

These elderly persons can benefit from care that maintains or upgrades their health or could specifically prevent an illness episode. Data from the author's research study are particularly persuasive for developing health policy for preventive care. One man, severely disabled by a stroke, was cared for by his wife and was ineligible for any public services because his needs were purely custodial. When she was absent for a short time and thus could not provide his care, severe deterioration resulted. That then allowed expensive nursing care services to be provided and reimbursed. Another patient, discharged from home care after her fractured hip healed, was severely depressed over her husband's recent death. Her depression and isolation led to decreased exercise, poor nutrition, and inadequate sleep, resulting in rehospitalization for pneumonia. Other case studies presented earlier demonstrate the great number of patients requiring expensive treatment and experiencing loss of health because reimbursable care was not available before the crisis.

The Flaw: Too Many Could Benefit

The major flaw in a proposal to provide preventive care is that nearly every elderly patient could benefit from preventive or maintenance care. Clearly, public funds cannot be expended just because someone would benefit. Objective criteria would be required to limit precrisis care to only those who otherwise would be institutionalized, thereby averting even greater public expenditures.

The outcome criterion for this group of patients would be either the achievement of health status that decreased the risk of institutionalization or a health status that showed continued need for services because the individual still was at risk for institutionalization. This group conceivably could remain eligible for services indefinitely. Reimbursement would continue only at a level that would be less costly to the public than nonhospital institutionalization (e.g., nursing home or congregate housing).

PROSPECTIVE REIMBURSEMENT PROBLEMS

A prospective reimbursement system has potential problems, too. The most important one is how to determine what efficiency will do to quality. Another is whether the savings generated by providers will be reinvested in the institution and in advanced services, forcing up the average cost of achieving care and of prospective reimbursement. A third is will patients be discharged prematurely to save money for the institution, and, if so, where will the needed additional home care resources come from? And fourth, will patient access be decreased for low paying DRG s? (Even with careful planning some DRG categories will have more potential for savings to institutions than others.)

The two elderly populations requiring home care services have criteria that are different as to outcomes but are similar for the determination of services needed. Each group would be assessed according to its functional limitations and the family type of resources available. Regardless of whether the ultimate goal were cure or prevention, the kinds of support needed would depend on self-care abilities or family assistance. The scope of required services, however, might differ substantially.

Those who had been hospitalized and were recovering from a specific episode of illness might well need continuing medical services: follow-up laboratory studies for the heart attack patient, specific dietary therapy for a new diabetic or one recovering from intestinal surgery, or radiation or chemotherapy for the person recovering from cancer. However, those who were at risk for health crisis because of their failing ability to care for themselves (weakness, visual deficits, arthritis deformities, or loss of a family member, for instance) might require only safety measures, custodial care, or more basic nutritional and ambulation assistance. Therefore, it would seem appropriate and cost effective for different kinds of agencies to provide care for different needs. Hospital-based home health agencies would provide home treatment for those discharged from the institution and community-based agencies would provide home services to those primarily in need of preventive and maintenance care.

Scope of Services

Hospital-based agenices have the services available in the institution that may be needed by patients recuperating at home: x-ray, laboratory services, pharmaceuticals, and consultation from physical, occupational, and speech therapists. In addition, the nurses who cared for these patients during the acute phase of their illnesses are available for planning, consultation, and perhaps for providing the home care on a rotating basis. Because all of these resources are used consistently and cost effectively for inpatients, they are available at lower cost and greater availability for those on home care who may use those services unpredictably or rarely.

Community-based home health agencies would not be required to provide the full scope of care because their primary clientele would be persons chiefly in need of nursing and support services. The one professional service required by all of these clients is nursing. Community-based agencies would provide professional nursing service, not only for assessment and outcome evaluation but also for nursing therapy in almost all instances.

Homemakers or home health aides might be needed on a regular basis by these patients, but their eligibility for public funding would rely on a professional determination of their at-risk status—a decision that cannot be the responsibility of a nonprofessional. In addition, the nurse for this population of patients is the consultant with other professionals regarding the provision of exercise regimes (physiotherapists), nutritional and dietary programs (nutritionists) or medication changes (physicians). Usually these professional consultations can result in a nurse-directed plan of care. Even when a patient has experienced a medical episode requiring these professional services, the convalescent (at-home) period usually can be managed in all of those areas without home visits by therapists other than nurses.

By eliminating the requirement that all home health agencies provide the full scope of eligible services, two important gains could result:

1. The cost of providing services would decrease because expensive and rarely used professionals would not have to be hired or contracted for by every agency.
2. Geographical areas poorly served by home health agencies would have increased access and availability because community-based agencies would be less costly and complex to establish.

Contact with Nurses

In addition to having nurses develop the plans for home services, there would have to be a way for patients or their families to contact nurses directly for care. The system now views nursing services as determined and referred by physicians. Access, cost effectiveness, availability, and legitimacy all would be enhanced if patients could go directly to nurses for the assessment and delivery of nursing services. Assessment visits and nutritional services have been reimbursed as administrative expenses, meaning that there was no evaluation of their effectiveness and that no value was placed on them as part of professional care. These services would have to come under the reimbursable framework.

Home visits now are reimbursable for physical, occupational, and speech therapists. Each of these specialists has a distinct service to offer but for patients well enough and stable enough to be at home, these professional services should be reimbursed only for a consultation and planning visit. Services that had been determined to be needed could be provided by nurses or support staff members who already were making regular visits to the home and who could incorporate the other professionally determined services into the same visit.

Even for the acutely ill hospitalized patients, nurses have been viewed as adequate to deliver basic physiotherapy exercises or nutritional counseling in the absence of the therapists (e.g., on weekends). Both physical and occupational therapy require home adaptation in most instances so the presence of those professionals in the home for planning services is essential. Speech therapy, however, does not require home adaptation, nor can it be shown to prevent institutionalization. That is not to say it is an unessential service; however, it might be more cost effective (and perhaps more beneficial in some instances) to provide those services only in a centralized area (not in individual homes) where one therapist could accommodate many more patients a day.

Care Visits: To Physician Offices or at Home?

Professionals who rarely make home visits under the current structure still are needed for service: the physicians. Many noninstitutionalized patients require medical care in their homes so an assessment or monitoring visit might be more worthwhile in the home setting. Patients can be assessed better when the stress and rigor of getting to the physician's office is obviated. Some who can survive safely and happily at home cannot make it to the physician's office because they are confined to a wheelchair or cannot ambulate in ice or snow, or their illness precludes any travel.

Physician home care should be reestablished and promoted under public reimbursement guidelines. Like the occupational and physical therapists, physicians would function as consultants in home services, providing the medical care planning. The nurse would be the primary provider of services and the coordinator of the various other professional plans of care. Physicians would participate by providing direction of the medical aspects of the plan. They primarily would provide information on and treatment for the patients' present illnesses. The most common are diabetes, high blood pressure, or other cardiovascular problems.

The home care plan, which centers primarily on the patient's functional status and overall health needs, obviously would be influenced by any current medical treatment. The physician would provide that information to be incorporated into the nurse's plan of care. For example, a patient might need nutritional guidance as well as assistance with dressing or housework. Information regarding the presence of diabetes, hypertension, or diverticulosis would influence the dietary plan, and a medical plan for arthritis or glaucoma would influence the self-help and safety routines.

The research study demonstrated, as noted earlier, that physician plans for home care services were inadequate half the time. Part of this severe deficit is attributed to the high number of referrals for home care being made by specialist physicians who either have no knowledge of patients' chronic medical conditions or who may know of them but do not report them. Therefore, it would seem an appropriate and safe measure to require that the medical consultation for home care services be provided by the patient's primary physician.

If the episode that required home care arose from a fractured hip, head injury, or other condition cared for by a specialist physician (e.g., orthopedist or neurologist), then information from both specialist and primary care physicians would be necessary. The open-ended referrals now used do not promote exchange of information regarding chronic medical conditions or resolved and currently untreated conditions (stroke, cancer, etc.). Perhaps a more explicit referral or information form for physicians is required.

The Role of the Family

The family resource is an important factor to be addressed in home care policy. While the number of elderly grows, resources are diminishing. Families whose assistance could be made available must have incentives to make the inevitable sacrifices required in caring for an elderly person.

A number of proposals need to be reexamined, including tax incentives or outright payment to families. Substitute family services also would have to be developed: homemakers, congregate or sheltered housing, and voluntary community services such as organizing the elderly to assist each other, or involving high school students in an adopt-a-grandmother (grandfather) venture.

All of these proposals require substantial resource development, either financial or from willing people. Neglect of such development would not simply lead to service deficits; it would result in unconscionable use of expensive institutional services—at public expense. In 1983, the Reagan administration proposed just the opposite of family subsidies: contributions from families would be required when elderly members received Medicaid-funded nursing home care. This would amount to a tax on those unfortunate enough to have frail, poor parents.

FUNDING CHANGES ESSENTIAL

Funding of home care must change to provide needed services and to promote equity in contributions by beneficiaries. Community-based home health agencies, primarily with nursing and support personnel, must be developed in rural and other underserviced areas. The Institute of Medicine study (1983) calls for increased services in rural and underserved areas. Funding for agency and service development has been unstable, unpredictable, and inadequate (Trager, 1980). If less complex agencies could be certified for preventive and maintenance services under public reimbursement programs (primarily Medicare), and if funding could be provided that assisted not only with initial development but also with continuing programs, access to care would be increased greatly. Increased access to basic home services could decrease inappropriate institutionalization, resulting in public savings even if home care developmental funds were provided.

Federally financed home care services are now funded primarily through payroll deductions, making the benefits an earned right. Additional home care benefits can be purchased through individual premiums and subsidization from general revenue taxes. In actuality, current workers pay for benefits for current retirees; the beneficiaries' contributions already have been spent to pay for earlier retirees, which somewhat affects the concept of "earned" benefits. More importantly, the tax on earnings is inequitable since high-income and low-income workers both pay the same dollar amount. On the basis of percentage of income, this means that the lower income workers are paying proportionately more for the same service eligibility. This inequity continues in the premium payments and in the copayment and deductible schemes contained in "competitive" health care payment proposals. To be more equitable, funding should be provided from general revenues (instead of employer-employee deductions), any individual contributions (copayments or deductibles) should be determined on a percentage of income/resources, and premiums should be eliminated (Davis, 1981).

The federal role in providing home care services undoubtedly faced changes, not only because of the movement toward decentralization but also because resources and needs were changing. One reason more of the funding of health services delivery was being turned over to the states was that the cost of the system had become exorbitant and unmanageable.

The states were reluctant to assume responsibility for the program because their resources were no better able to fund the system. The federal program also had been shown to be wasteful and inequitable, another reason for making changes. And finally, the elderly population was growing and its health needs were mounting proportionately, along with the continuing need to be able to pay hospital bills.

The federal role should continue to include funding. Without a national perspective and commitment, health care for the elderly would fall victim to more parochial interests and short-term funding. Financing must be provided from taxes in a more equitable way than the wage deductions system. Program costs can be contained by further efforts to deliver cost-effective services in lieu of institutionalization. Resource development, for both facilities and personnel, must be a national effort to assure access and availability. Health outcomes must be set at the national level; the elderly everywhere should have services aimed at the same goal—prevention of institutionalization. Standard setting for quality and appropriateness also belongs at the national level in order to assure the elderly everywhere that care delivered under cost-containment guidelines still will meet their true needs in a satisfactory manner.

NEW STATE AND LOCAL FUNCTIONS

A complementary role can be envisioned for state and local governments in the delivery of federally funded health services. Kinds of services needed for the elderly to achieve common health outcomes might differ substantially from state to state in the country. For some, maintaining safe independence and preventing institutionalization would require homemaker services; for others, the key service needed could be meals-on-wheels; and for still others, it might be the services of a nurse on a regular basis, or transportation to health care, or supervised living in congregate housing. Each provider receiving federal reimbursement for health care for the elderly would have to justify how expenditures directly furthered the aim of preventing institutionalization.

It is clear that congregate housing, homemaker services, or any of the other needed services cannot be developed ad hoc on the basis of a single individual's needs, and yet federal reimbursement for health care was only for individual claims—no money was available for service development.

One way to provide services needed on a state or local basis is to develop community-based agencies on a capitation basis. An agency could be funded based on the number of elderly to be cared for, and the services to be developed would be those most needed by the target population. Part of the outcome evaluation for the agency funding would be a report on utilization and health outcomes of those services for the people served. In this way needed services could be developed, with agency accountability for their use.

The local role in federally funded health services thus would include the determination of structure and process of care, important variables when individualizing services to a given population. The aggregate health and health-related social benefits would be available from one agency and under the aegis of one funder/evaluator. Feder, in her research on Medicare and the policy process (1977), points out that one of the fallacies in the nation's health policy is the idea that social and health needs can be separated and treated in isolation from one another. Although not specifically addressing the family, Feder's analysis helps explain the poorly understood role of the family in health care policy.

Welfare policy traditionally has funded social benefits whereas health policy tends to finance illness care. This uneasy dichotomy does explain why "family care," which incorporates both social and health care, is difficult to characterize or to find alternatives for in its absence. Whether services are labeled "health care" or "social care" makes little difference in the amount of money needed from the national budget to meet those needs.

HOW BEST TO SPEND THE DOLLARS?

It may be time now to experiment with combinations of services to see how best the federal dollar can be spent to keep the elderly independent and out of institutions. Preventing medical episodes and maintaining health are ways of doing just that, and a combination of social and health benefits may be needed to achieve those outcomes.

A single entry system is necessary to assure that patients will not receive inadequate or duplicate services. The community-based agency would be the appropriate entry level for home health services. Existing community resources are poorly coordinated, with expensive duplications and glaring omissions of services. All the federal programs serving the elderly (Titles XVIII, XIX, and XX of the Social Security Act, P.L. 89-97, and P.L. 89-73, the Older Americans Act) have separate entry level qualifications, offer duplicate services, and all omit coordination of care and lack quality and outcome measurement of patient status (DHEW, 1979).

There is little traffic between levels of care, and indeed patients confined to nursing homes rarely return home again to live with the help of home care services. Home care patients tend not to go to nursing homes; they usually wait until they are sick enough for a hospital, and nurses assist them in this. If the home care system were more responsive to a greater variety of needs, institutionalization surely could be decreased further. To be more responsive will require extensive efforts to coordinate and monitor services already in the community as well as to develop ways of providing substitutes for families and for social programs that no longer are sufficient in number or resources to serve the elderly.

These recommendations have been made with the expectation that regulatory policy in home health services will continue to evolve. Although home health services accounted for only 2.6 percent of total Medicare payments in 1982, reimbursement for them was increasing at a higher rate than for other Medicare services. The alternative to greater regulation to control these trends is to let the market forces determine use and, as many researchers have written, there is no free market in health care; the providers determine use (Kavaler, 1980; Somers, 1978; Vladeck, 1980).

Kavaler notes that the power and influence of physicians, and the unequal ability of the neediest to get services, make continued regulation a necessity. In an article on the future of regulation, she notes that the 1980s should see a reallocation of resources based on needs. Bice (1980) and Klarman (1980) call for more demonstration research as a prelude to more regulation, so that more will be known about what processes work before an attempt is made to mandate any of them.

Vladeck makes a convincing case for continuing regulation in health services. He believes that this is the only way to assure access and services to those who need them and that the government must be accountable to taxpayers for use of their money in providing health care. Mechanic (1981), like Kavaler, believes health regulation will tend toward allocation of funds to providers to assist defined populations, with the range of services and level of coverage mandated by government, but with great discretion on actual care offered to any one individual, and with some freedom for providers to determine priorities.

Changes that are needed in home care policy threaten the provider beneficiaries of existing policy—primarily the physicians. Needs of patients, and the public pressure for cost containment, however, present powerful arguments for those changes.

REFERENCES

Berkman, L., & Syme, S. Social networks, host resistance and mortality. *American Journal of Epidemiology,* November 1979, *109*, 186-204.

Bice, T. Social sciences and health services research. *Milbank Memorial Fund Quarterly,* Spring 1980, *58*(1), 201-216.

Brook, R., & Lohr, K. Quality of care assessment: Its role in the 80s. *American Journal of Public Health,* July 1981, *81*, 681-682.

Callahan, J. Responsibilities of families for their severely disabled elders. *Health Care Financing Review,* Winter 1980, 29-48.

Carr, W. Presentation to Doctoral Seminar "Measuring unmet health needs." Columbia University School of Public Health, March 1980.

Davis, K. *Competition in Health Care.* Paper presented at the convention of the American Public Health Association, Los Angeles, November 1981.

Feder, J. Medicare implementation and the policy process. *Journal of Health Policy, Politics & Law,* Summer 1977, *3*(2), 173-189.

Hammond, J. Home health care cost effectiveness; An overview of the literature. *Public Health Reports,* July-August 1979, 305-311.

Home care in New York State. Albany, N.Y.: Home Care Association of New York State, May 1979.

Home health: The need for a national policy to better provide for the elderly. Department of Health, Education, and Welfare, Report to Congress, December 1977.

Home health care services: Tighter fiscal controls needed. Department of Health, Education, and Welfare, Report to Congress, May 1979.

Institute of Medicine. *Nursing and nursing education: Public policies and private actions.* Presentation to National Academic Press, Washington, D.C., 1983.

Kane, R., & Kane, R. Care of the aged: Old problems in search of new solutions. *Science,* May 16, 1978, 913-918.

Kavaler, F. Regulation of health care prospects for the future. *Public Health Policy,* 1980, *1*(3), 230-240.

Klarman, H. Health services research and health policy. *Milbank Memorial Fund Quarterly,* Spring 1980, *58*(1), 201-216.

Levenson, I. Some policy implications of the relationship between health services and health. *Inquiry,* Spring 1979, 9-12.

Mechanic, D. Some dilemmas in health care policy. *Milbank Memorial Fund Quarterly,* Winter 1981, *59*(4), 1-15

Mundinger, M., & Jauron, G. Developing a nursing diagnosis. *Nursing Outlook,* February 1975, 94-98.

Mundinger, M. *Autonomy in nursing.* Rockville, Md.: Aspen Systems Corporation, 1980.

New York State Legislature, Long Term Health Care Program, Chapter 895, 1977.

Pegels, C. *Health care and the elderly.* Rockville, Md.: Aspen Systems Corporation, 1980.

P.L. 89-73, the Older Americans Act (1965).

P.L. 89-97, Social Security Amendments of 1965 (Medicare, Medicaid).

P.L. 95-210, the Rural Health Clinic Services Act of 1977 (the Medicare and Medicaid Amendments).

Somers, A. The high cost of health care for the elderly: Diagnosis, prognosis, and some suggestions for therapy. *Journal of Health Policy, Politics & Law,* Summer 1978, *4*(2), 163-180.

Trager, B. *Home health care and national policy.* New York: Hawthorne Press, 1980.

Van Dyke, F., & Brown, V. Organized home care. *Inquiry,* June 1972, 3-16.

Vladeck, B. *Unloving care.* New York: Basic Books, Inc., 1980.

Weissert, W. *Effects and costs of day care and homemaker services for the chronically ill elderly.* NCHSR, February 1980.

Wolfe, S. Unmet health care needs and health care policy. Presentation at the American Association for the Advancement of Science symposium on *Health Goals and Health Indicators,* Washington, D.C., 1977.

Wolfe, S. Presentation to Doctoral Seminar, Columbia University School of Public Health, February 7, 1980.

Index

About the Author

MARY MUNDINGER is Director of the Graduate Program in the School of Nursing at Columbia University. She graduated from the University of Michigan, is a Family Nurse Practitioner and received the Doctor of Public Health in Health Policy from the Columbia University School of Public Health. She has written extensively on professional issues in nursing, including primary nursing, nursing diagnosis, and the role of nurse practitioners.

Her book, *Autonomy in Nursing,* published by Aspen Systems Corporation in 1980, won the AJN Book of the Year Award in 1981 and is now in a second printing. Dr. Mundinger, her husband, and their four children live in Rye, New York.